SMART MEDICINE for MENOPAUSE

Hormone Replacement Therapy and its Natural Alternatives

SANDRA CABOT, MD

AVERY
a member of Penguin Putnam Inc.

The information and procedures contained in this book are based upon the research and the personal and professional experiences of the author. They are not intended as a substitute for consulting with your physician or other health care provider. The publisher and author are not responsible for any adverse effects or consequences resulting from the use of any of the suggestions, preparations, or procedures discussed in this book. All matters pertaining to your physical health should be supervised by a health care professional.

The excerpt on page 170 is from *Always a Woman* by Kaylan Pickford, published by Bantam Books in 1982. Reprinted by permission.

Cover designers: William Gonzalez and Rudy Shur
In-house editor: Amy C. Tecklenburg
Typesetter: Bonnie Freid
Printer: Paragon Press, Honesdale, PA

Library of Congress Cataloging-in-Publication Data

Cabot, Sandra.
    Smart medicine for menopause : hormone replacement therapy and its natural alternatives / Sandra Cabot.
        p. cm.
    Includes bibliographical references and index.
    ISBN 0-89529-628-4
    1. Menopause—Popular works. 2. Menopause—Hormone therapy.
I. Title.
RG186.C23 1995
612.6'65—dc20   95-7001
                                                         CIP

Printed in the United States of America.

20 19 18 17

CONTENTS

PREFACE

The terms "menopause" and "change of life" often arouse feelings of fear, dread, uncertainty, and confusion. Yet even though menopause is one of the greatest physical milestones in a woman's life, it does not have to be traumatic or painful.

At around the age of fifty years, a woman's biological clock stops ticking, signaling the loss of fertility and the loss of the sex hormones estrogen and progesterone. Vitally important questions are raised by the loss of these parts of her identity. Questions such as:

• How will I feel—mentally, physically, and sexually—without sex hormones?

• Will I age more rapidly without estrogen in my body?

• Will I still be able to function efficiently and compete with younger women in the workplace?

• Will my husband lose interest in me and take a younger lover?

• Will I lose my femininity and look masculine?

• If I have a premature menopause, can I still have a baby?

• Will I get osteoporosis?

Read on, and all these questions—and many more—will be answered. This book is your menopause handbook and will serve as a lifeline to guide you through this often awesome and bewildering time of life. It discusses all your options in a simple and clear way, and will leave you fully informed. Most of all, it will take the fear out of menopause and put you back in the driver's seat.

A woman passing through menopause and beyond needs to know about all her options, and is likely to have many unanswered questions about them. For example:

• Do I need to take hormones in the form of hormone replacement therapy?

• Can I use natural hormone replacement therapy instead of the old-fashioned synthetic hormones?

• If one type of hormone replacement therapy doesn't help me, can I take hormones in other forms?

• What is the difference between hormone pills, injections, patches, creams, implants, and suppositories?

• If I don't want hormone replacement therapy, what else can I do to cope with the symptoms of menopause?

• Is there anything I can do to slow down the aging process?

With the information in this book, you can master menopause and emerge with your vitality, femininity, sexuality, and peace of mind intact. Indeed, in many cases the change of life can be a change for the better.

Sandra Cabot, M.D.

Chapter 1

MENOPAUSE IN A NUTSHELL

My fifty-four-year-old patient had sat for hours on the bus, all the way from an isolated country town called Lightning Ridge, to seek help. She flopped into the chair on the other side of my desk with a desperate and exhausted look in her eyes. She told me that male doctors had no time to listen to her woes and merely threw up their hands, saying that she was "just getting on in years." She said that life was cruel for women going through menopause, and that she felt like a sexless, emotionless "it." Indeed, she felt as if she had been cheated. She certainly did *not* want to hear, "That's life; it's just part of getting older."

I have heard countless tales like this and—perhaps because I am a woman, too, and not just a doctor—I can empathize with the plight of these frustrated women. But we do not have to passively suffer the problems of menopause. There are real, safe, and simple solutions for today's menopausal woman—solutions to help us recapture our former mental and physical well-being and to slow down the ravages of time on our minds and bodies.

Women are still occasionally told that menopause is part of Mother Nature's design, and that they should accept it as gracefully as their mothers did. In fact, however, our mothers may have died—as women still die today—from some of the long-term complications of menopause. Fortunately, today's woman has a wide array of choices available—including hormone replacement therapy, counseling, nutritional supplements, dietary modification, and general medical treatment—to help ensure that her passage to midlife and beyond is a fruitful and pleasant voyage.

1

WHAT IS A HORMONE?

Before we deal with menopause in depth, it is important to understand what hormones are and how they function in the body. Hormones are body chemicals that carry messages from one part of the body to another. They are made in specialized glands called endocrine glands (see Figure 1.1) and are circulated in the blood to specific body cells where they make their presence felt.

The thyroid gland manufactures thyroid hormone, the adrenal glands manufacture the adrenal hormones epinephrine (also called adrenaline) and cortisone, and the ovaries produce the sex hormones estrogen and progesterone. These are just a few of the many hormones required to keep our cells functioning in harmony.

Hormones are concerned with controlling the chemistry of cells. They determine the rate at which our cells burn up food and release energy. They also determine whether cells produce milk, hair, secretions, enzymes, or other metabolic products.

Hormones are extremely potent molecules. In some cases, less than one millionth of an ounce of a hormone is sufficient to exert an effect. Individual hormone molecules are far too small to be seen, even under a microscope.

Hormones can be likened to chemical "keys" that turn vitally important metabolic "locks" in our cells. The turning of these locks stimulates activity within the cells of the brain, intestines, muscles, genital organs, and skin. Indeed, all our cells are influenced to some degree by these amazing hormonal keys. (See Figure 1.2.)

Without the hormonal keys, the metabolic locks on our cells remain closed and the full potential of our cells is not realized. Imagine a corporation where the employees are unable to communicate with the president and are left to do their own thing. The corporation would lack any unified direction and would be unable to grow. This type of chaos is what would happen in your cells without hormones.

After hormones have completed their tasks, they are either broken down by the cells on which they have acted or are carried to the liver for breakdown. The resulting compounds are then excreted or used again to manufacture new hormone molecules.

CAN HORMONES RUIN YOUR LIFE?

An imbalance in or lack of hormones can shatter your life. Among other things, hormones are vital for making you sexually responsive, passionate, and sensitive, and for sustaining mental drive.

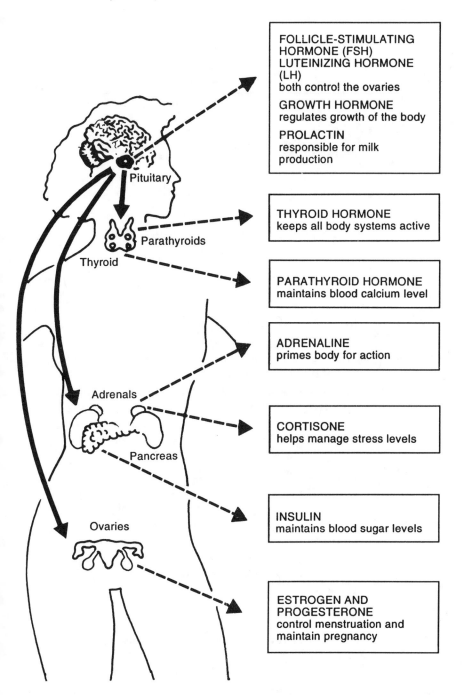

Figure 1.1 Endocrine Glands and Their Hormones

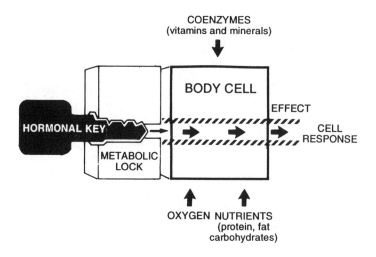

Figure 1.2   How Hormones Affect Cells

According to consultant gynecologist John Studd of the Meno-pause Clinic at Kings College Hospital in London, England, adequate amounts of sex hormones keep women "out of the orthopedic wards, the divorce courts and the madhouse."[1] Before hormone replacement therapy (HRT) became available, a significant percentage of meno-pausal women suffered a severe midlife crisis that was called, in medical terminology, *involution melancholia*. This old-fashioned term describes the shrinkage of mind and body that can occur without the presence of sex hormones. Some women became so profoundly de-pressed that they were institutionalized for the rest of their lives.

Hormones control many aspects of human behavior and emotions, and help to make you a mentally competent, functional person. They are involved in the system of *psychoneuroendocrinology*, which is the complex interaction of the mind, the nerves, and the endocrine (hor-monal) system. We are only beginning to understand that many mental illnesses, such as manic-depressive illness and schizophrenia, have a chemical basis.

The brain has its own natural "happy hormones," called endor-phins, that act on the pleasure centers in the brain and help us cope with pain and emotional turmoil. If these brain hormones become depleted, you may suffer a deep and gloomy depressive illness. Imbalances of various hormones can create such devastating and insidious signs of malfunction as personality changes, panic attacks, agoraphobia, poor memory, insomnia, frigidity, reduction of sex drive, obesity, blood sugar problems, allergies, and inflammation—and this list is far from exhaustive.

The medical specialty in the treatment of hormonal disorders is called *endocrinology*. We can now accurately measure the levels of the vast majority of the body's hormones with blood tests, and we are able to replace many of these hormones if the various glands of the endocrine system fail to manufacture them in adequate amounts. This is how the term *hormone replacement therapy* (HRT) came to be.

Hormones—they can make you or break you, make your life heaven or hell, and be responsible for untold miseries. However, thanks to modern biotechnology, genetic engineering, pharmacology, and nutritional medicine, we can now control our hormones. This is truly a powerful medical development, with implications as momentous as the discovery of penicillin.

In this book you will discover the influence of hormones on your mental and emotional state, your ability to succeed, your sexuality and appearance, and the rate at which you age. You will be amazed by the way hormones influence your menstrual cycle, your immune system, and your chances of getting osteoporosis, cancer, and cardiovascular disease.

HOW ATTITUDES HAVE CHANGED

The attitude of doctors towards menopausal women has changed—slowly—over the last century. In 1850, the most famous gynecologist of the day, a Frenchman called Colombat, preached to the medical profession that "all women who have reached this critical period of life should withdraw themselves from the vicissitudes of atmospherical influences, lest they promote plethoric accumulations [congestion with blood] in their regenerative organs, which should henceforth be left in a state of inaction." He was obviously out of touch with women, to say the least! He was virtually saying that once you're menopausal, you should retire from many of life's passions and pleasures. If men had to experience the discomforts of menopause, we'd probably have had effective treatments for them centuries ago!

Today, many experts regard the postmenopausal phase of a woman's life as a potential "hormone deficiency disorder," which is a far cry from the negative attitude of doctors such as Colombat. Women's lives are changing, both physically and socially. Our average lifespan has increased from a mere fifty years at the beginning of the 1900s to approximately eighty years today. By the year 2050, it will be ninety-five years or more, and thereafter should continue to increase, according to some predictions. The average woman today spends 40 percent of her life in a postmenopausal state, so you can understand why the long-term problems of menopause and the postmenopausal years have assumed huge medical, social, and economic significance.

WHAT CAUSES MENOPAUSE?

The word *menopause* means the cessation of menstrual bleeding, which is a sign that estrogen production has fallen to very low levels. This happens when the ovaries, the female reproductive organs, become unable to manufacture the sex hormones estrogen and progesterone. Menopause can thus be called ovarian failure.

Why Do the Ovaries Fail?

This is the million-dollar question. The human female is the only creature known to outlive her sex glands and reproductive capacity. One may well ask, "Why us? Did Mother Nature go haywire? Or are we simply living longer than God intended?"

Even though we may wish it didn't happen, the fact is that our ovaries simply run out of follicles (eggs) at around the age of fifty years. It is the follicles within the ovaries that produce the vast majority of estrogen and all of the progesterone.

Are the Ovaries of Any Use After Menopause?

The ovaries do have an important function after menopause because they can still produce very small quantities of estrogen and significant amounts of testosterone for a period of approximately twelve years. Thus, the ovaries of a menopausal or postmenopausal woman are certainly not dead, dying, or useless organs. This is why the issue of whether these organs should routinely be removed in menopausal women undergoing hysterectomy remains complex and controversial. If you are faced with this decision, it is wise to obtain several expert opinions.

After menopause, the adrenal glands continue producing—and indeed, may increase their production of—hormones that are then converted into estrogen in a woman's adipose (fat) tissue. This adrenal gland production of estrogen may continue for up to twenty years after menopause. The amount of estrogen produced this way varies, depending on the amount of body fat an individual has and on the health of her adrenal glands. Heavier women, who have more adipose tissue, tend to have higher total levels of estrogen than thin women. This is probably the reason that heavy women often appear to age more slowly than very thin women. There is no benefit in being underweight as you pass through the menopausal years.

The amount of the hormone testosterone produced by your ovaries is very significant and continues to be so in the postmenopausal years. The ovaries are probably a more potent source of testosterone than the adrenal glands are, and so contribute greatly to sexual desire and enjoyment during the postmenopausal years. In some women, the relatively greater amount of testosterone produced by the postmenopausal ovary may lead to an increase in facial hair, thinning of the hair on the scalp, and shrinkage of the breasts.

Do We Have a Simple Test for Menopause?

The menopausal ovary, being devoid of eggs, is unable to manufacture significant amounts of the female sex hormones. If a blood test is done to measure the levels of estrogen and progesterone, they will be found to be at low levels. In menopausal and postmenopausal women, blood estrogen levels (which are measured in the form of estradiol, the most active form of estrogen) are generally less than 54.4 picograms per milliliter (pg/mL). (A picogram is a minuscule amount used as standard laboratory measurement.)

The function of the ovaries is under the control of the pituitary gland, which is situated at the base of the brain and acts as the master controller for the many hormonal glands in the body. The pituitary gland is very sensitive to the hormonal output of the ovaries, and it begins to react when the ovaries fail to pump estrogen and progesterone into the bloodstream. The pituitary gland is not at all happy with the failure of the menopausal woman's ovaries. It quickly starts to pump out large amounts of a hormonal messenger called follicle-stimulating hormone (FSH), which travels to the flagging ovaries to try to stimulate them back into action. Alas, the stubborn ovaries have closed up shop forever and, despite the hormonal pleas and wooing from the pituitary gland, the ovaries remain dormant. Meanwhile, the pituitary gland cannot comprehend that the ovaries are unable to respond to its advances and, in a futile attempt to reawaken them, it continues to pump ever-increasing amounts of FSH into the bloodstream. This achieves nothing as far as the ovaries are concerned, but it does provide a useful diagnostic test your doctor can use to assess whether you are menopausal. Typically, blood FSH levels are quite high if you are menopausal, usually between 40 and 200 milli-international units per milliliter (mIU/mL). This is ten to fifteen times higher than the normal level for women not yet approaching menopause.

These blood tests can be very useful if you are suffering from many and vague symptoms for which your doctor can find no obvious cause. Symptoms such as chronic fatigue, rheumatic aches and pains, anxiety, depression, and poor libido may be due to a relative deficiency of estrogen and progesterone, which is not uncommon in the years leading up to menopause. This time of life is called the *premenopause*, and though it typically occurs when a woman is in her late forties, it may start at any time after the age of thirty-five. It is often associated with a change in the pattern of the menstrual cycle, with menstrual bleeding becoming erratic—less or more frequent, or heavier or lighter in amount. During the premenopausal years, blood tests to measure the levels of estrogen, progesterone, and follicle-stimulating hormone may be able to pinpoint a relative deficiency of estrogen and progesterone. If a deficiency is identified, appropriate hormone replacement therapy can be taken to correct it.

During one of my country trips, a premenopausal woman came up to speak with me after I had given a lecture. She had been complaining of hot flashes, anxiety, panic attacks, headaches, neck aches, and a total loss of libido. She had seen several doctors, who asked her if her menstruation was still regular. As soon as she replied that she menstruated at monthly intervals, their verdict was that she could not possibly be suffering from a deficiency of estrogen and that her symptoms must be due to stress. She was given prescriptions for sedatives and anti-inflammatory drugs and was told to rest more and cease reading women's magazines. This woman was very angry at her doctors' attitude and was made to feel that she could not cope with the so-called normal phases of life.

A blood test to measure hormonal levels is a simple and relatively noninvasive procedure. It may also be appropriate to try a course of natural hormone replacement therapy for at least three months to see if these premenopausal symptoms can be alleviated. Such treatment can be dramatically effective and often prevents or eliminates the need for sedatives, antidepressants, painkillers, and anti-inflammatory drugs in premenopausal women.

Some women are told not to worry about their hormones until they stop menstruating completely; once this occurs, they can return to the doctor. But by this stage you may have suffered for years—which in this day and age is no longer necessary—and even your friends will be able to pronounce you menopausal! You won't need a doctor to make the diagnosis.

Many body cells need estrogen to maintain their normal function. For example, the cells of the vagina, bladder, breasts, skin, bones, arteries, heart, liver, and brain all have estrogen receptors and require estrogen to stimulate these receptors for normal cellular function. The loss of the three sex hormones—estrogen, progesterone, and testosterone—may be associated with an increase in the incidence of heart attacks, high blood pressure, and osteoporosis, as well as an increased risk of cancer and abnormalities in the brain's chemistry.

THE FIRST SYMPTOMS OF MENOPAUSE

The signs and symptoms that signal a deficiency of estrogen can be divided into acute signs (those that occur immediately) and chronic signs (those that occur over the long term). The symptoms that most women notice first are the acute symptoms, including hot flashes, aches and pains, vaginal dryness, bladder problems, dry and aging skin, sleep difficulties, and a variety of emotional changes.

Hot Flashes

Probably the most telltale sign of all is the onset of hot flushes, or, as they are more commonly called, hot flashes. You may feel hot and flustered even though everyone else is cool, calm, and collected—and complaining bitterly when you open windows and turn off the heat.

Hot flashes occur because the body's thermostat, situated in the area of the brain known as the hypothalamus, does not function at all well when it is deprived of estrogen. One minute you may be cold and shivering; the next minute you may feel like an inferno, with an irresistible desire to pull off all your clothes and bedding. One patient of mine told me that her nocturnal hot flashes kept her husband warm all night, so that he no longer needed to turn on the electric blanket. Another patient found her hot flashes extremely embarrassing. They caused her glasses to fog up, and the younger men she worked with thought she was getting hot and excited about them!

Nearly 80 percent of menopausal women are troubled by hot

flashes, and in 70 percent of this group the flashes will occur, on average, over a period of five years. Hot flashes vary in severity and may be associated with heart palpitations, dizziness, and strange crawling or itching sensations under the skin.

Aches and Pains

Another possible acute symptom of estrogen deficiency is an increase in bodily aches and pains. For instance, your headaches may become more frequent or severe, your joints may ache, your back and neck may ache, and you may begin to suffer from various rheumatic aches and pains.

Vaginal Dryness

The vaginal tissues are very sensitive to the effects of estrogen deficiency. More than 50 percent of menopausal women are troubled by vaginal dryness and failure to achieve adequate lubrication during sexual intercourse. This causes discomfort or pain during sex and, in severe cases, may result in some bleeding from the fragile mucous membrane lining the vagina. Without the strengthening effect of estrogen, the vagina may become more prone to infection by candida (yeast) and bacteria, which may result in vaginal discharge, itching, and burning.

Over the long term, atrophy (a general shrinkage) of the vagina, the vaginal opening, the vulva (the vaginal lips), and the clitoris may occur. This can have a devastating effect on a woman's sexuality. Fortunately, as we shall see later in this book, there are treatments available that are extremely effective for preventing these changes.

Bladder Problems

The tissues of the bladder are also sensitive to estrogen deficiency. Some menopausal women complain of a frequent and/or urgent desire to pass urine, urge or stress incontinence (a reduced ability to control the passage of urine), a reduced bladder capacity, and an increased susceptibility to cystitis (bladder infection). Needless to say, any of these problems can cause discomfort and/or embarrassment. Fortunately, they can be overcome by a combination of pelvic floor exercises, hormone replacement therapy, and/or nutritional measures.

Dry and Aging Skin

Both the superficial and deeper layers of the skin on our faces and bodies are sensitive to estrogen, as are the collagen fibers that criss-cross in the deeper skin layers. Without estrogen, the skin becomes thinner and more fragile, more prone to developing discolorations and broken capillaries ("spider veins"), and less capable of retaining moisture. The skin is more prone to dehydration and irritation, and collagen depletion results in a more rapid appearance of wrinkles.

Poor Sleep

Estrogen deficiency can adversely affect sleeping patterns, so that difficulty going to sleep or early-morning waking can set in. The problem may be associated with, or made worse by, the occurrence of hot flashes during the night. We know that insomnia is related to estrogen deficiency because sleep disorders are often helped by hormone replacement therapy, especially if the problem is associated with hot flashes. Studies have shown that taking estrogen increases the proportion of sleep time spent in the dreaming phase. Many women find that taking estrogen improves poor memory and decreases irritability. This may be due in part to estrogen's beneficial effect on sleep.

Emotional Changes

Mental and emotional changes are common at the time of menopause. The most common complaints are depression and anxiety. Personality changes may occur, with rapidly changing moods, irritability, loss of confidence, and panic attacks occurring in women who had none of these problems before menopause. An inability to cope, both mentally and emotionally, is often more poignantly evident in career women who occupy high-profile positions of great responsibility than it is in women who lead less stress-filled lives. Some women say that they feel numb and can no longer muster any passion or *joie de vivre*. If this occurs on a physical level, a woman may experience a total loss of libido and, in extreme cases, she may become completely unresponsive sexually.

And Then There's . . . Your Mental Attitude

Your mental attitude is a powerful factor in coloring your personal experience of menopause. Estrogen deficiency does not affect all

Estrogen Level Score Chart

The chart below lists acute symptoms that are characteristic of an estrogen deficiency. It is adapted from a menopause questionnaire devised by Professor Chris Nordin of the Institute of Medical and Veterinary Science at Adelaide University in Adelaide, South Australia.

Rate the severity of each menopausal symptom, as you experience it, and then add up your total score for all the symptoms listed. Use the following scale to rate the severity of your symptoms:

Absent – 0; Mild – 1 point; Moderate – 2 points; Severe – 3 points

Symptom	Score
Depression and/or mood changes	_____
Anxiety and/or irritability	_____
Feelings of being unloved or unwanted	_____
Poor memory and concentration	_____
Poor sleeping patterns (insomnia)	_____
Fatigue	_____
Backache	_____
Joint pains, arthritis	_____
Muscle pains	_____
Increase in facial hair	_____
Dry skin and/or sudden development of wrinkles	_____
Crawling, itching, and/or burning sensations in the skin	_____
Reduction in sexual desire	_____
Frequency of or burning sensation with urination	_____
Discomfort during sexual intercourse	_____
Vaginal dryness	_____
Hot flashes and/or excessive sweating	_____
Lightheadedness or dizziness	_____
Headaches	_____
Total score	_____

If your total score for all of these symptoms is 15 or more, then it is likely that you are suffering from a deficiency of estrogen.

If your score is around 30, your body is probably crying out for estrogen. This can be confirmed or refuted by a simple blood test to check your levels of estrogen and follicle-stimulating hormone.

If you are on hormone replacement therapy, it is an interesting exercise to score your symptoms of estrogen deficiency both before and on a weekly basis for two months or so after starting HRT. After that, computing your score every three to four months will provide a useful self-check to see whether your hormone replacement therapy is adequate. However, you should not decide to alter your dosage based on the results of this questionnaire without first consulting with your doctor.

---

women in a negative way. Indeed, some women simply sail through menopause with no emotional changes. Some women find that the cessation of hormonal highs and lows associated with monthly menstrual cycles makes their menopause a time of tranquility and composure. It is therefore dangerous to stereotype menopausal women, or we could all be brainwashed into having a midlife crisis!

The common emotional changes associated with menopause are not always caused by estrogen deficiency alone. There may be numerous psychosocial stresses in your life, such as having adolescent children, caring for elderly parents, coping with the altered self-image that comes with aging, dealing with your husband's midlife crisis, or experiencing "empty-nest syndrome." All these stresses can take an emotional, mental, and physical toll, especially on the caring, giving type of woman who may find that she is continually supporting others but is receiving no support or praise in return. If this true for you, I strongly recommend that you indulge in some well-deserved self-nurturing—take a vacation, arrange for regular massages, practice tai chi, or do something really adventurous!

You may be amazed that the lack of estrogen can cause such a vast array or diversity of possible symptoms. The reason for this is that receptors for the hormone estrogen are found on most of the body cells, from the brain to the skin, genital organs, and bones. To assess your own symptoms of estrogen deficiency, use the Estrogen Level Score Chart on page 12.

I often think back to how it was sixty years ago for women passing through these powerful physiological and emotional changes. In those days, there was little understanding and even less sympathy for the symptoms that women suffered, usually alone and stoically. Thankfully, we no longer live in an era of confusion and ignorance, and women should expect to have their cases heard by sensitive and caring doctors. Once the cause of your symptoms is understood, they can be treated scientifically and effectively. This is a great relief. Women no longer have to feel like helpless victims of the loss of their sex hormones and of the aging process.

Chapter 2

THE LONG-TERM CONSEQUENCES OF ESTROGEN DEFICIENCY

The life expectancy for women in Western societies today is eighty to eighty-five years. The fastest growing segment of the population in these countries consists of people over fifty-five years of age, and most of these people are women. In the United States, there are currently more than 100,000 women over the age of 100.

When a woman becomes menopausal, she can anticipate another thirty to forty years of life. This means that she will spend around 40 percent of her life span in a postmenopausal state—in other words, without sex hormones in her body. Wow! That sounds fairly dramatic, profound, and perhaps—for the majority of women, who love feeling and acting like women—a little frightening.

The long-term effects of estrogen deficiency vary among different women, owing to genetic, psychological, and environmental factors. In other words, some women will suffer from effects of estrogen deprivation, while others will not, and this individuality is obvious to a doctor specializing in this area. Overall, the loss of estrogen results in a higher risk of osteoporosis, cardiovascular disease, and sexual dysfunction in postmenopausal women.

However, there is much that you and your doctor can do to prevent or offset this higher risk.

VAGINAL ATROPHY

Five years after menopause, most women will have some thinning, dryness, and atrophy (shrinkage) of the vagina, unless they take estrogen replacement therapy. I have seen quite a few women in their sixties and seventies who have continued to have active and fulfilling sex lives. For the increasing number of women in their seventies and eighties who want to be sexually active, vaginal atrophy is a real concern. However, for many women, the biggest problem is not deciding whether to be sexually active, but finding a partner, as on average, men don't live as long as women do.

CARDIOVASCULAR DISEASE

Forty percent of American women will suffer from heart disease or a stroke. Up to the time of menopause, women enjoy a certain amount of protection against cardiovascular disease (diseases of the heart and blood vessels) compared with their male counterparts. Indeed, the incidence of heart attacks in women is only one third as great as the incidence in men. Unfortunately, after menopause, women begin to lose this relative protection from heart attacks and strokes, so that by the age of seventy-five, a woman's risk of developing these problems is similar to that of a man.

Menopause and Cardiovascular Risk

Why do women become more prone to cardiovascular disease after menopause? The most important factor appears to be the loss of estrogen in the body, which results in unfavorable changes in blood cholesterol levels. Not only do overall cholesterol levels tend to rise, but the level of low-density lipoproteins (LDL, or "bad cholesterol") goes up, while that of high-density lipoproteins (HDL, the so-called "good cholesterol") goes down. After menopause, this imbalance in cholesterol results in an increase in atherosclerosis (the process of blockage and hardening of the arteries), especially in women who smoke, who are obese, and/or who have sedentary lifestyles.

Early menopause is bad news for your cardiovascular system. Women who lose the function of their ovaries before the age of forty have a greater risk of heart disease than women who go through menopause when they are ten years older. The good news is that large-scale population studies, such as the Framingham Heart Study, have proven that estrogen replacement can restore a favorable balance in cholesterol levels.

The risk of cardiovascular disease can be reduced by approximately 50 percent by taking estrogen at or soon after menopause. A landmark nurses' health study with 48,000 subjects—the first prospective study of women on hormone replacement therapy—found breakthrough results for heart disease.[1] After ten years, it was found that there were half as many cardiovascular deaths and heart attacks among women who took estrogen after menopause as there were among women who had never used estrogen.[2] It is important to note, however, that this applies only if natural (not synthetic) estrogens are used. To put it in a simple way, if you took two large populations of women and gave one group natural estrogen for twenty-five to thirty years after menopause, but gave no natural estrogen to the other group, the women who took estrogen would have half the risk of heart attack as compared with the others. This is because estrogen reduces total cholesterol levels, increases the proportion of the so-called "good cholesterol," and prevents cholesterol from being deposited in the walls of the arteries.

The reduction of strokes by hormone replacement therapy appears to be more modest, but it is still significant. A recent study of 23,088 Swedish women showed that postmenopausal estrogen replacement therapy can reduce the overall risk of stroke by 30 percent.[3]

We know for sure that estrogen alone is good for your blood vessels and heart, but we are not sure if taking synthetic progesterone in addition to estrogen (as is now commonly done) reduces the benefits of estrogen on your cardiovascular system, particularly if you take estrogen and progesterone for many years. We are still searching for the ideal progesterone.

Your risk of cardiovascular disease is not determined only by the loss of estrogen. Other risk factors are equally important—and sometimes more important—as determinants of cardiovascular disease. These include smoking, high cholesterol levels, a family history of cardiovascular disease, high blood pressure, obesity, lack of exercise, a high-fat diet, and a diet that is deficient in raw foods, fish, and liquids such as water and fresh juices. (See Chapter 6 for ways to minimize these risk factors.)

The Good News About the Long-Term Use of Hormone Replacement Therapy

As we continue to live longer and longer, the possible long-term effects of estrogen deficiency become more and more important. In other words, how might the lack of estrogen in your body affect you twenty-five to forty years after menopause?

The inaugural scientific meeting of the Australian Menopause Society, held in Brisbane in September 1989, came up with some brain-snapping facts. A study of 8,841 women in a southern California retirement community found that women who had used estrogen replacement therapy had a significantly reduced risk of death from all causes compared with women who had never taken estrogen. Much of this was due to a marked reduction in the death rate from heart attacks in women on estrogen. The lowest death rate was seen in long-term users of estrogen.[4]

At this meeting, Professor Brian Henderson of the University of Southern California at Los Angeles said that taking natural estrogen led to a 50-percent reduction in the risk of heart disease and stroke, giving women an additional 4.2 years of life on average. Another benefit of natural estrogen cited at the meeting was a lower death rate from some types of cancer. In particular, hormone replacement therapy appears to reduce the risk of cancer of the ovary by up to 40 percent.[5]

The main benefit of estrogen in prolonging life comes from its ability to reduce heart disease. This becomes clearer when we look at the total relative risk of death from various causes for women over fifty, summarized in the famous nurses' study cited on pages 16–17. This study found that there is a 31-percent overall risk of death from heart disease, a 2.8-percent risk of death from breast cancer, a 2.8-percent risk of death following hip fracture, and a 0.7-percent risk of death from uterine cancer.[6]

So overall, in the long term, we may be better off taking natural estrogen than not taking it. Still, many women, and many doctors, are reluctant to use adequate doses of estrogen for sufficient periods of time. Perhaps this is because they still think of HRT as it used to be twenty years ago, when large doses of synthetic estrogen were taken without the proper balance of progesterone. This resulted in a higher incidence of uterine cancer, blood clots, and high blood pressure. Unfortunately, it also left the impression that all HRT is controversial. This is not so. The natural estrogens of today are so safe that they cannot realistically be compared to the superhuman doses of synthetic estrogens that were given years ago. Provided you undergo all the necessary preliminary tests and examinations, the use of natural estrogen should add years to your life, as well as greatly improving its quality.

OSTEOPOROSIS

Dr. Frederick S. Kaplan, a professor of orthopedic surgery at the

University of Pennsylvania, wrote in 1987, "If hypertension is a silent killer, osteoporosis is a silent thief. It insidiously robs the skeleton of its banked resources, often for decades, until the bone is weak enough to sustain a spontaneous fracture."[7]

Osteoporosis has also been called the "silent epidemic." It currently afflicts one in every three postmenopausal women in Western society—which is a little depressing, isn't it? But there is some good news. If women take the right precautions early enough, this insidious bone-weakening disease can be prevented. None of these precautions are too hard, and like most things, they're up to us.

Osteoporosis results from the abnormal loss of calcium from the bones, which causes them to weaken and become susceptible to fracture (breakage). It was once thought that osteoporosis was simply a normal part of the aging process and that it should be accepted gracefully because, after all, it was just a manifestation of Mother Nature's design. We now know this is untrue. Osteoporosis is a disease, and it can be avoided in most cases. Nowadays, no woman should have to suffer its debilitating effects.

Some epidemiologists predict that by the year 2050, the world will be full of little old ladies, one third of them suffering from osteoporosis. I feel that this is unduly pessimistic, as doctors now know how to prevent this disease. I believe that by the year 2050, we will see the good results of preventive medicine reflected in a much lower incidence of osteoporosis than is currently the case.

Today, osteoporosis is very common; by the age of sixty, one in four women living in the Western world develops a significant degree of bone loss. Most women in the early stages of osteoporosis are free of symptoms—so what we're dealing with is indeed a silent epidemic.

By the age of seventy-five, one quarter of all women sustain a fracture of the hip. Nearly one third of the women who fracture a hip die within six months. Osteoporosis is thus the twelfth leading cause of death in America. Every year in the United States, some 200,000 hip fractures occur, 85 percent of them in women. Furthermore, approximately 60,000 of these women die each year. The osteoporosis epidemic increased during the 1970s and 1980s, and appears to be increasing still; indeed, if the tide is not stemmed, we could be looking at a half-million hip fractures annually by the year 2000.

By now you are probably shaking in your boots, feeling that it would be easier to avoid death and taxes than osteoporosis. But don't despair. By following a few simple guidelines, you can prevent osteoporosis. The first step is to assess your risk factors.

Risk Factors for Osteoporosis

There are a number of definite risk factors that tell if you are likely to develop osteoporosis. Among them are your race, your body type, and lifestyle factors such as diet, exercise, and the use of tobacco and certain medications. (To get an idea of your own risk of developing osteoporosis, see the Osteoporosis Risk Chart on page 21.)

Race

The first risk factor for osteoporosis is your racial background. If you are Caucasian or Asian, your chances of developing osteoporosis are higher than they would be if you were black. African-American women tend to achieve greater bone density prior to menopause and experience a slower rate of postmenopausal bone loss.

Body Build

Your body build can be a risk factor. Women with excess weight and those of normal weight are less likely to suffer from osteoporosis than thin women—so there are some benefits in being a little cuddly, after all! This is because hormones produced by the adrenal glands are converted into estrogen in the fat, or adipose, tissue. This is a significant source of estrogen after the ovaries have failed. Being thin, even underweight, may be glamorous for your image, but it is likely to increase your chances of developing osteoporosis. If your bones are very fine—in other words, if your skeletal frame is small—you will be even more likely to develop osteoporosis.

Smoking

Another major risk factor for osteoporosis is smoking. Smoking is bad news for your skeleton because it reduces the production of female hormones by the ovaries, thereby increasing the loss of calcium and other minerals from the bones. This is yet another good reason for women who smoke to kick the habit.

Medications

Taking certain medications may predispose you to osteoporosis. If you swallow large amounts of antacids containing aluminum over a long period of time, this may increase the loss of calcium from your

Osteoporosis Risk Chart

The chart below lists some of the factors that affect your chances of developing osteoporosis. Circle the appropriate scores in the right-hand column and add the numbers up at the bottom to score your own risk for osteoporosis.

Risk Factor	Score
Amenorrhea (lack of menstruation) for:	
6–12 months	1 point
12–24 months	2 points
2–5 years	3 points
5–10 years	4 points
10 years or more (unless you have had a hysterectomy and are receiving adequate hormone replacement therapy, in which case score 0)	5 points
First menstrual period after the age of 17 (late puberty)	1 point
Long-term use of cortisone	5 points
Family history of osteoporosis	3 points
Small, fine-boned frame	2 points
Calcium deficiency during adolescence and/or while nursing a child	2 points
Tobacco use	1 point
Lack of weight-bearing exercise	2 points
Excessive exercise, especially if it leads to amenorrhea	2 points
Caucasian or Asian racial background	1 point
Excessive consumption of protein, salt, alcohol, caffeine, soft drinks	1 point
Overactive thyroid (excess thyroxine)	1 point
Total score	_____

If your total score is under 5 on this scale, you have a low risk of developing osteoporosis.
If your total score is 5 to 8 points, you have a moderate risk of developing osteoporosis.
If your total score is 9 or more points, you have a high risk of developing osteoporosis.
The most accurate way to determine your risk is to have a bone mineral density test done at the time of menopause (see page 27). A bone mineral density test is able to determine the density and therefore the strength of your bones. If your bones are dense, then they are more resistant to fracture. A bone mineral density test should be a routine screening test for all menopausal women. It should be considered as essential as a cholesterol test, Pap smear, or mammogram.

bones. It is preferable to take antacids that are free of aluminum—ask your pharmacist about suitable brands. Avoid using aluminum cooking utensils, as they give you a regular supply of unwanted aluminum. Excessive amounts of aluminum may interfere with calcium metabolism, thereby increasing the risk of osteoporosis.

Cortisone-type drugs also rapidly accelerate the loss of calcium from the bones. If you must take cortisone preparations, you should take them only when absolutely necessary and in the lowest possible dose for the shortest possible time.

Diet

The vital role of diet in the development of osteoporosis was evident to me when I vacationed in Miami Beach in the early 1970s. Miami Beach was then a retirement haven for upper- and middle-class Americans, and one would have expected to see a population of happy, relaxed older women enjoying the good life of the American Dream. On the contrary, I was shocked to see older women who seemed to move slowly and without vitality, many of whom had a "dowager's hump"—a curvature of the spine creating a rounded hump in the upper back—which is a classic sign of osteoporosis. They seemed older than their years as they plodded along, the curves of their spines forcing them to look at their feet rather than at the sunny skies of Miami.

Ironically, many of these women had brought osteoporosis upon themselves, while living in a land of plenty, because of their long-term consumption of excessive amounts of animal protein, phosphorus (largely found in processed foods), salt, and sugar. A diet like this increases your risk of osteoporosis because it increases the excretion of calcium in the urine and/or disturbs the balance of calcium in the body, so that calcium passes out of the bones and into the blood. We do not need large amounts of animal protein for good health. Many Americans consume 100 to 120 grams of protein from animal sources (meat, fish, dairy products) daily, which is more than double what they need. To prevent the loss of calcium, we should consume less than 50 grams of animal protein daily. One three-ounce portion of fish, meat, cheese, or chicken has 21 grams of protein, so you can see how easy it is to consume more than 50 grams.

What I was seeing in the early 1970s is now a statistical phenomenon often talked about during conferences on osteoporosis. In Western societies, osteoporosis is becoming a much bigger problem, afflicting ten times as many women as it did in the 1950s and often appearing at a younger age. Experts agree that the reasons must be our lifestyle, diet, and increasing life span. Women who drink excessive amounts of alcohol and caffeine are also increasing their risk of osteoporosis, although a modest social intake (for alcohol, no more than four to five alcoholic drinks per week; for caffeine, the equivalent of six to seven cups of coffee per week) does not appear to increase the rate of bone mineral loss.

There are two types of osteoporosis that affect the bones in different ways. Both types of osteoporosis can be influenced by a poor diet.

Bones consist of two primary layers: the *cortical bone*, the dense, compact outer layer, and the *trabecular bone*, the more spongy, porous inner layer (see Figure 2.1). Type-1 osteoporosis causes a loss of trabecular bone and is mainly due to a lack of sex hormones, specifically estrogen and androgens. Type-2 osteoporosis causes a loss of cortical bone and is mainly due to deficiencies of calcium and/or vitamin D.

The amount of estrogen produced by your body is affected by the amount of calories you consume. If you are a chronic dieter and consume a very low calorie diet, and especially if your menstrual periods are infrequent and light, you may suffer from a premature estrogen deficiency, which can lead to type-1 osteoporosis.

You are more likely to suffer from type-2 osteoporosis if your diet is specifically lacking in calcium and/or vitamin D. The recommended daily allowance (RDA) for calcium is 800 milligrams for

Periosteum —

Cortical bone —

Trabecular bone —

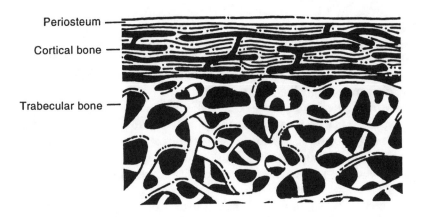

Figure 2.1   The Structure of a Long Bone
Bones are composed of a dense outer layer, the cortical bone, and a spongier inner layer, the trabecular bone, both contained within a tough, fibrous membrane called the periosteum.

premenopausal women and 1,000 milligrams for menopausal and postmenopausal women. It is alarming to learn that *three quarters of all women fail to consume these RDAs.* This sets the stage for the development of type-2 osteoporosis. By eating plenty of calcium-rich foods, you can ensure that you get at least the RDA of calcium each day. (See Chapter 6 for information about food sources of calcium).

Your intake of calcium during adolescence and when you are in your twenties is crucial in determining your peak bone mass (the ultimate mass that your bones achieve). Today, many adolescent girls are reducing their peak bone mass by stringent dieting and excessive exercise. This will increase their risk of developing osteoporosis later in life.

The ratio of calcium to other minerals in the diet is also important. The ratio of calcium to phosphorus, for example, should be 2 to 1. Yet the modern-day Western diet contains so much phosphorus that the balance has tipped in favor of *phosphorus* by 4 to 1. This excess of phosphorus can speed up loss of calcium from the bone. You should aim to reduce the amount of high-phosphorus foods in your diet by avoiding products whose labels include ingredients such as phosphoric acid, sodium and potassium phosphate, polyphosphate, and pyrophosphate. Generally, phosphorus and its derivatives are found in processed or canned meats; processed cheeses; any processed foods that are laden with artificial preservatives, flavorings, and colorings; packaged cookies and pastries; fizzy soft drinks; and packaged breads and cereals. By now you are probably wondering where your nearest health food store is, as many of the products found at your local supermarket or convenience store are loaded with phosphate additives.

The mineral magnesium is important in helping your body to utilize calcium. If you increase your intake of calcium, you should raise your intake of magnesium as well. The ideal calcium-to-magnesium ratio is 2 to 1; therefore, if you consume 1,000 milligrams of calcium a day, you need 500 milligrams of magnesium daily. If you take these minerals in supplement form, it is possible to obtain tablets containing both calcium and magnesium in the correct ratio of 2 to 1.

The antioxidant vitamins C and E are important as well. They are necessary for the manufacture and maintenance of the tough, fibrous collagen in our bodies. Collagen gives our bones flexibility, making them less brittle and more resilient in the face of sudden stresses.

A deficiency of vitamin D may also predispose you to developing osteoporosis. Vitamin D deficiency has been found in 30 percent of postmenopausal women with bone deterioration.[8] Unlike other vitamins, vitamin D is actually a hormone that is synthesized in your skin when it is exposed to direct sunlight. However, many women now choose to avoid the sun as much as possible because of its aging effects on the skin. You can also obtain vitamin D from liver, especially fish liver; fatty fish such as halibut, mackerel, and salmon; butter; eggs; and vitamin-D-enriched milk. Women who are likely to suffer a vitamin D deficiency include those with food-absorption or digestive problems and intolerances to any dietary fat, as well as those who get no exposure to sunlight. If any of these applies to you, you should consult your doctor for a blood test to measure your level of vitamin D and determine whether you need vitamin D supplements, and, if so, at what dosage. Generally speaking, a daily supplement of 400 international units of vitamin D is adequate and safe.

Other nutrients that help calcium to keep your bones strong and healthy are boron, vitamin K, copper, zinc, manganese, and silica. A good multiple vitamin and mineral tablet should contain all of these nutrients.

Exercise

Women who do not get regular weight-bearing exercise are at far greater risk of developing osteoporosis than those who do. Weight-bearing exercise is *not* the same thing as weight-lifting. It is any type of exercise that involves movement in the upright position, so that body weight is transmitted through the spine, pelvis, and legs to the ground—in other words, exercise in which the force of gravity acts vertically downwards on the skeleton. Ideally, this exercise should involve muscular contraction. Examples of suitable weight-bearing exercise include thirty minutes daily of walking, jogging, aerobics, or yoga. It is best to choose a form of exercise that you can adopt as a lifestyle. However, you should be aware that too much exercise can reduce body fat excessively, causing estrogen levels to drop. In extreme cases, menstruation may cease. If this happens, it reflects a dangerously low estrogen level—and increases your risk of developing osteoporosis. Moderation in exercise is the key.

Heredity

Genetic factors are important in determining how dense your bones will become. Consider yourself to be at a higher than average risk if your mother, grandmother, or sister has developed osteoporosis. Fortunately, you can help to offset this increased risk by adopting a healthy lifestyle and eating a high-calcium diet.

Menopause—THE Most Important Risk Factor

The loss of the hormone estrogen at the time of menopause is the major cause of osteoporosis. If women did not go through menopause, their incidence of osteoporosis would be closer to that of men—that is, it would be approximately twenty times lower. The earlier the menopause and the longer a woman spends in the postmenopausal state, the greater her chances of developing osteoporosis. Women who experience premature menopause are at particular risk. But the women *most* at risk are those who have had their ovaries surgically removed, especially if this is done before they reach the age of forty-five, and who have never received adequate hormone replacement therapy.

If you have a combination of several risk factors, your chances of developing osteoporosis are multiplied. You should therefore do everything possible to remove these risks and decrease your chances of developing the disease. For example, if you are thin, eat a poor diet, smoke cigarettes, drink alcohol excessively, and reach menopause before the age of forty-five, you would be a prime candidate for developing osteoporosis. Fortunately, many if not most of these risk factors are things that you can control.

The Signs of Osteoporosis

Unfortunately, in many cases, the first sign of osteoporosis is the fracture of a bone, particularly in the wrist, hip, or spine, after minimal damage or trauma. To avoid this painful outcome, you should be aware of the signs that may indicate the earlier stages:

• A gradual reduction in height. If your dresses and slacks seem to be getting longer, that may be a warning sign.

• A stooping of the spine and rounding of the shoulders. This happens when the normally square-shaped spinal vertebrae gradually collapse into triangular wedges. If this is allowed to continue, you may develop a hump on your spine, below the neck, that is rather disparagingly called a "dowager's hump."

• General aches and pains in the bones may signal early osteoporosis, so remember, all that aches is not necessarily arthritis. Be wary of accepting anti-inflammatory arthritic medication or painkillers without first having tests done for osteoporosis.

• If the texture of your skin changes, rapidly losing its thickness and suppleness at the time of menopause, then it is more likely that collagen loss is occurring in the bones. It is the loss of collagen fibers in the dermal layer of the skin that causes sudden wrinkling and loss of texture. Brittle nails and deterioration of the teeth may also be a clue. According to experts at Kings College in London, the development of osteoporosis is due partly to a loss of collagen in the bones, which causes them to become excessively brittle. The loss of collagen in the bones is often mirrored by a loss of collagen in the skin.

Is There a Reliable Test for Osteoporosis?

Doctors have a test called a bone mineral density test that can accurately predict your chances of developing osteoporosis. The bone mineral density (BMD) test measures the concentration of minerals in your bones to determine how strong and resistant to fracture the bones are.

Ideally, all women should have a BMD test when they pass through menopause, *not* several years later, as bone mineral loss can be rapid in the first five years after menopause. Ask your doctor for a referral to a medical facility experienced in administering the BMD test. Ideally, such a facility should be equipped with the latest lunar DPX-L bone densitometer machines, which utilize dual energy x-ray absorptiometry (DEXA) technology. Measurements of bone density should be made in the spine and hips. By the way, ordinary x-rays are not an accurate test for osteoporosis.

The BMD test takes fifteen to twenty minutes to perform and does not involve any injections, drugs, or discomfort. It is accurate to within one half of one percent and emits less radiation than a dentist's x-ray. It really is an ideal test that your doctor can use to monitor your bone density at regular twelve- to twenty-four-month intervals over many years and give you peace of mind.

Figure 2.2 illustrates the acceleration of bone loss that often occurs when a woman passes into the estrogen deficiency zone of menopause. The dotted line represents the bone fracture threshold, which is the point at which bone mineral density becomes so low that a bone may fracture under the slightest stress. In the unfortunate women whose bones reach this threshold, the fracture of a hip may occur simply as a result of jumping out of bed and putting all the weight on one hip; a vertebral compression fracture in the spine can be caused by sitting in a car traveling over a rough road. Indeed, if your bone density crosses the fracture threshold, you become a virtual "china doll."

In Figure 2.2 you can see that the time zone around menopause, represented by the shaded column, is a crucial time corridor where the loss of bone mass can be greatly accelerated. Indeed, because of the loss of estrogen during this time, a rapid bone-loser can lose a large amount of her total bone mass. More than 50 percent of the total amount of bone that is lost in the postmenopausal years is usually lost in the first seven to ten years after menopause. A new blood test to identify your risk of osteoporosis should become available within the next few years. It is based on the fact that researchers have identified a gene that determines bone strength or density.

Preventing Osteoporosis

Osteoporosis afflicts over 10 million of the 30 million American women over the age of fifty, and results in more than 1 million bone fractures annually. The overall cost of treating and caring for Americans with osteoporosis is around $10 billion a year.

The current epidemic of osteoporosis in women aged sixty and above reflects the fact that ten years ago, there was no accurate test to discover the very early stages of this disease. Consequently, women came for medical attention only when they had developed bone fractures or humping of the spine. And unfortunately, at this

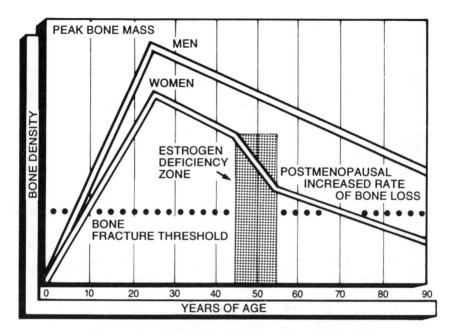

Figure 2.2   The Increasing Risk of Bone Fracture
Associated With Menopause

The diagram above shows the change in average bone mass for women, by age; the dotted line represents the point at which bone density is so low that a fracture may occur with only the slightest stress. Notice that bone loss is most rapid between 45 and 55 years of age—the period around menopause.

advanced stage it is difficult to put back the calcium that has leached out of the bones. But the good news is that we can prevent the loss of calcium from from the bones if treatment is begun early, at the time of menopause—not ten years later.

Hormone Replacement Therapy

Hormone replacement therapy is the most effective method of preventing osteoporosis. Ideally, HRT should begin when the deficiency of sex hormones first becomes apparent—usually at the time of menopause or, in some women, in the premenopausal years. Many studies have shown HRT to be the most effective treatment for the maintenance of bone size and strength and for the prevention of bone fractures. HRT must be taken for fifteen to twenty years to prevent osteoporosis effectively.

After three years of treatment, women who receive estrogen ther-

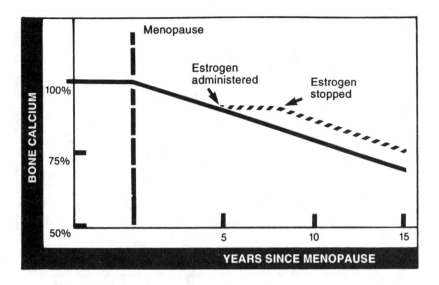

Figure 2.3   The Effect of Estrogen Therapy on Bone Mineral Loss

In this diagram, the solid line shows the rate at which the bones lose calcium in the years after menopause; the dotted line shows the effect of estrogen therapy. It demonstrates that estrogen therapy can virtually halt the loss of calcium from the bones, although when estrogen is discontinued, calcium loss resumes.

apy have about 10 percent more bone than those not on HRT. Figure 2.3 shows the effect of estrogen therapy in slowing the rate of bone loss. One in three women is what we call a "fast bone-loser." In such women, estrogen replacement is able to slow the rate of bone loss so that the fracture threshold is never crossed.

HRT is a powerful tool against osteoporosis because it not only reduces the loss of minerals from the bone, but slows the loss of collagen from the skeleton as well. It also slows the loss of collagen from the deeper layers of the skin, and it is thought that this effect slows the rate of aging of the skin. It seems that HRT is good not only for your inner layers but also for your outer layer!

Osteoporosis can cause the bony vertebrae of the spine to become weak and spongy, and their once-rectangular solid forms to be crushed into triangular wedges. These are called compression fractures (see Figure 2.4). Compression fractures cause a loss of height, a protruding abdomen, and a curved posture, with compression of the spinal nerves that causes sharp shooting pains in the spine and limbs.

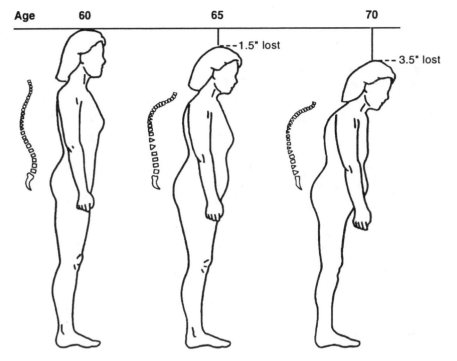

Figure 2.4 Compression Fractures of the Spinal Vertebrae

Compression fractures occur when the normally rectangular vertebrae, weakened by osteoporosis, are crushed into triangular wedges, causing a reduction in height and changes in posture.

Currently, one in four American women over the age of sixty-five has one or more spinal compression fractures.

A loss of bone mass also commonly occurs in the hips, and without preventive treatment, 50 percent of postmenopausal women are at risk of a hip fracture by the age of seventy-five. Taking estrogen replacement therapy for fifteen years after menopause postpones the age of high fracture risk to ninety years. Currently, the average life span for American women is eighty-five years, so HRT in effect enables the majority of women to escape fractures. Women who use estrogen therapy have a 60 percent lower risk of osteoporotic fractures than women who do not.[9] As women continue to live longer, they may need to take HRT for longer periods; the ideal solution would be to reprogram the ovaries to pump out estrogen indefinitely.

In addition to estrogen, some progestogens have worthwhile ability in reducing bone loss. This provides another reason for combining estrogens and progestogens in HRT prescriptions.

Calcium Supplementation

Calcium plays a role in building up your peak bone mass and reducing the bone loss associated with aging and menopause. Bone fracture rates in the elderly are reduced when adequate calcium intake is maintained. Professor Chris Nordin of Adelaide University in South Australia is a brilliant authority on calcium metabolism. He recommends that you take 500 milligrams of calcium daily if you consume dairy products regularly, and 1,000 milligrams daily if you do not. Table 6.3, in Chapter 6, will enable you to make sure that your diet and calcium supplements provide you with at least 1,000 milligrams of calcium daily. It has been found that fewer than 40 percent of menopausal women have an adequate daily intake of calcium.

Calcium supplements are best taken last thing at night, just before you go to bed, because it is during sleep and when your stomach is empty that blood calcium levels fall. To replace it, parathyroid hormone dissolves precious calcium from your bones. By taking calcium before sleep, you can prevent this.

Anabolic Steroids

Anabolic steroids are male hormones (natural and synthetic) that are well known for their infamous role in competitive sports, yet few people know that they are often used to help women with established osteoporosis. The rationale for their use is that menopausal women with high blood levels of testosterone lose bone more slowly than women with lower testosterone levels. The role that anabolic steroids play is not clear, but they have been shown to help prevent bone loss and may even bring about some degree of bone gain in cases of established osteoporosis.

Anabolic steroid tablets and injections may be very useful for women with osteoporosis who are unable to take estrogen. You should be aware, however, that these drugs can cause oily skin, pimples, fluid retention, and weight gain, as well as an increase in facial hair, deepening of the voice, and increased libido. As a result, some women who try them discontinue use of them. On the other hand, many women find that these drugs reduce musculoskeletal pains and greatly increase vitality.

Regular Daily Exercise

Exercise is a vitally important strategy for preventing osteoporosis. As discussed earlier in this chapter, the right kind of activity is a weight-bearing exercise such as walking, jogging, aerobics, or yoga, done for thirty to forty minutes, every day. You should avoid overexercising, however (see page 26).

Treatments for Osteoporosis

Unfortunately, there is no cure for osteoporosis. There are, however, a number of medical treatments available that show some promise for treating the disease.

Etidronate

This drug reduces the resorption (loss) of bone and is most useful for women with severe osteoporosis and those unable to take estrogen. It can restore the strength of demineralized bone and reduce the frequency of spinal fractures.[10] Etidronate it is sold by prescription under the brand name Didronel. It is currently used primarily as a treatment for Paget's disease (another bone disease that chiefly afflicts the elderly) and certain metabolic disorders, rather than as a treatment for osteoporosis. If you think you might be interested in trying etidronate, I suggest you consult with a bone specialist, preferably one who has a particular interest in osteoporosis, who is experienced in using this drug and may be comfortable treating you with it.

Calcitonin

Calcitonin is a natural hormone that is extracted from salmon or eels. It delays bone loss both during and after menopause, even in older women with established osteoporosis. It is sold under the brand names Calcimar, Cibacalcin, and Miacalcin.

At present, calcitonin is expensive and must be taken by daily injection (a home injection kit is available). A nasal spray form is currently under research, and hopefully will be available soon. This would make it much easier to use, and it could become a very useful alternative for the prevention and treatment of osteoporosis, especially for many women who are unable to take estrogen replacement therapy.

Calcitriol

Calcitriol (vitamin D3) is the active form of natural vitamin D. It is sold under the brand name Rocaltrol. A large scientific trial in women with postmenopausal osteoporosis showed that over a three-year period, calcitriol reduced the incidence of new spinal fractures by 70 percent and that of other bone fractures by 50 percent.[11] Although this is encouraging, other studies have found it has less benefit for the bones in the limbs, while confirming that it strengthens the spine. If you take calcitriol, you must not also take calcium supplements unless you check with your doctor first.

All of these treatments are encouraging, but the fact is that modern medicine still does not have the ability to reverse severe established osteoporosis. What doctors *can* do extremely well is to prevent osteoporosis by the use of treatment in the premenopausal, menopausal, and postmenopausal years. Do not be lulled into a false sense of security; start taking precautions in your premenopausal years, and you won't be robbed by the silent thief in the years ahead.

Preventing osteoporosis is important not only for our individual well-being, but also for the sake of society as a whole. The percentage of older persons in our population is increasing, and while today's affluent society has the resources to care for the health of these people, this may not always be so. Epidemiologists estimate that by the year 2025, the percentage of persons under fifteen years of age will have gone from approximately 35 percent (in 1901) to approximately 19 percent, while the percentage of persons over sixty-four years of age will have increased from approximately 4 percent to approximately 16 percent. The smaller number of younger persons will find it increasingly difficult to support the health of the larger number of older persons, both financially and socially. To avoid the high cost to society of providing health care for our aging population, we must use the tools of preventive medicine while we are in midlife.

Moreover, women generally outlive men, and a large number of widows will spend around a decade without their partners. If they cannot maintain mental, emotional, and physical health, they may be forced into nursing homes and institutions, where care is expensive and their health may deteriorate further.

I do not want to sound like a prophet of doom, however. Rather, I want to help you realize that you are likely to have a better menopause and postmenopause if you take active responsibility for your own mental and physical health. This means ensuring that your doctor assesses your risk for cardiovascular disease, osteoporosis, cancer, and degenerative diseases at the time of your menopause. If such problems are found at this early stage, they can be corrected and further deterioration prevented.

We know that if hormone replacement therapy is given for ten to fifteen years after menopause, we achieve a large reduction in the incidence of heart attacks, stroke, and bone fractures. Theoretically, such reductions in these common diseases that afflict older women should become more evident as hormone replacement therapy is continued beyond the age of sixty-five.

Looking at these statistics, you may be convinced that every menopausal woman should have HRT. However, this is not necessarily the case. Each woman is unique. For example, some menopausal women have no troublesome symptoms and are not at risk of cardiovascular disease or osteoporosis, as determined by a bone density test and total physical examination. Such low-risk women have no medical need for HRT. However, they may still decide to take it for personal reasons, such as the desire to maintain a more youthful appearance or a more fulfilling sex life.

Whether you decide to take HRT or not, it is wise to begin a lifestyle and nutrition program for preventive health care. Strategies like getting regular exercise and increasing your intake of low-fat, high-calcium, and high-fiber foods, as well as raw fruits and vegetables, are probably more important than the decision to take hormone replacement therapy alone. Full details on diet, nutritional supplements, and exercise for midlife and beyond will be discussed in Chapters 6 and 7.

I believe that we can become what we visualize ourselves to be. Give yourself positive affirmations; tell yourself that you will be strong, energetic, and mentally switched-on as you age, and work toward these goals every day in a practical way. Don't let anyone convince you that your health must decline with age. I have witnessed thousands of women who have improved with age, and who have actually started to look and feel younger once they began using the miraculous healing tools of modern and naturopathic medicine together with a healthy lifestyle.

Chapter 3

YOUR VISITS
TO THE DOCTOR

I recommend that all sexually active women visit their doctors annually for a complete physical examination. In this way, problems can be detected early, and we all know that prevention is better than cure. It is essential that you develop a good rapport with your doctor and feel comfortable about expressing your deepest concerns. Don't worry if it takes a little searching to find a doctor you feel at ease with.

An annual checkup is important even if you do not want hormone replacement therapy or other prescription treatments. If you are more interested in natural health care alternatives, you may want to find a doctor who specializes in, or at least is knowledgeable, about these areas. Some women prefer to visit both a doctor and a natural therapist, so that they can have the best of both worlds. This is a good idea, although unfortunately it may be a little too expensive for some.

Women who do not experience unpleasant symptoms at menopause may be reluctant to consult a doctor, or may think there is no reason to, because they have no need or desire to have any "treatment." It should be emphasized that menopause is *not* a disease, and it is important not to medicalize it by taking an overly interventionist approach. However, the risk of certain serious diseases rises rather sharply at this time of life, so regular physical examinations become more important than ever for the maintenance of your good health.

Whatever your situation, a good doctor should take your individual perspective and needs into account. In addition, because the changes that menopause produces in your body are gradual, both you and your doctor should be aware that your needs and feelings may change over time. There is no need to rush into any treatment or to feel pressured by a doctor; the goal is to stay in tune with your body and work with your doctor to optimize your health.

This chapter will give you a good idea of what to expect at those all-important medical checkups.

YOUR FIRST VISIT

I suggest you consult a gynecologist or a doctor who has a special interest in women's health when you first experience premenopausal symptoms. If you are one of those lucky women who experiences no premenopausal symptoms, you should visit a doctor once you realize that menopause is taking or has taken place. Your first visit should be around thirty to forty minutes long, thus allowing time for a full history and physical examination.

Your History

Before deciding what medical treatment, if any, is appropriate for you, your doctor must take a medical history and perform a full physical checkup and a battery of tests. At the time of menopause, your ovaries, adrenal glands, and adipose (fat) tissue may still produce enough sex hormones to keep you feeling well. In the ten years after menopause, your levels of sex hormones will gradually decline, and at some point you may feel a desire to try hormone replacement therapy. Your doctor would then want to know if there are any risk factors in your family history that could influence the decision to begin HRT. For instance, if you have a strong family history of breast cancer—if first-degree relatives (a mother, sister, or daughter) have had the disease, and especially if it was diagnosed before menopause—your doctor would be more conservative about giving you estrogen replacement. Conversely, if you have a family history of osteoporosis or cardiovascular disease, your doctor would be more likely to advise you to take estrogen replacement on a long-term basis, as this would reduce your chances of following in your relatives' footsteps.

Particular attention should be paid to your menstrual pattern. If you have had irregular bleeding, or any bleeding after regular menstruation had stopped for twelve months, you will need to have a curettage of the uterus or a hysteroscopy performed. Curettage of the uterus is a procedure in which the lining of the uterus is scraped away so that it can be examined under a microscope for the presence of abnormal cells. Hysteroscopy is a relatively new procedure in which the doctor passes a flexible telescope through the opening of the cervix into the inner cavity of the uterus to view the uterine lining; if abnormal tissue is seen, this can then be biopsied (sampled). Both of these are usually outpatient (same-day) procedures performed under general anesthetic. They are done to rule out the possibility that bleeding is being caused by abnormal tissue, especially uterine or cervical cancer. If such a condition is discovered, urgent treatment, usually surgery, will be required. If physical conditions are ruled out as a cause of irregular bleeding, we can say that the bleeding is due to hormonal changes.

If you are interested in taking HRT, a previous history of gynecological cancer is very significant. If you have had successful treatment of a previous cancer of the ovaries or cervix, then HRT should not be a problem. However, if you have had endometrial cancer (a cancer of the inner lining of the uterus)—even if the cancer was treated successfully—taking estrogen could theoretically stimulate a recurrence. Check with the gynecologist and/or the oncologist (cancer specialist) who treated your cancer before making a decision regarding HRT.

Your past history of other medical problems is also worth scrutinizing. A woman's risk of developing cardiovascular disease rises significantly at menopause, so detection and treatment of high blood pressure, heart disease, or blood clots, for example, becomes important at this time. In addition, if you have any of these problems, special care is needed making a decision about HRT, specifically in deciding the type of HRT that is best for you. Your doctor will also want to know about your lifestyle and daily habits, as well as your expectations and needs concerning your sex life. Ideally, before starting HRT, if you smoke, you should stop; if you lead a sedentary life, you should begin to exercise regularly; and if you are overweight, you should slim down.

Your doctor will also quiz you about your menopausal symptoms, such as hot flashes, to assess your level of estrogen deficiency. Why not make it easier for your doctor by taking along your completed estrogen deficiency score chart? (See page 12.)

If you are enjoying an active and fulfilling sex life, you can optimistically anticipate that it can continue through menopause. HRT in particular can be helpful in ensuring a lasting quality to this pleasure. It definitely helps with vaginal and vulval lubrication and with the ability to achieve a satisfying orgasm, as well as preventing shrinkage of the breasts, uterus, vagina, and clitoris. Most women want to remain sexually active way beyond menopause.

Finally, your contraceptive needs should be discussed, because until your menstrual cycles stop completely, you may still be ovulating, at least occasionally. This means that there is theoretically still a slight risk of pregnancy. And even if you decide to take HRT, that does not guarantee 100-percent protection against pregnancy, as hormone replacement is not as effective in suppressing ovulation as the oral contraceptive pill. If you are premenopausal or in the very early stages of menopause, when there is still a chance of ovulation, you have a number of contraceptive choices.

If you prefer oral contraceptives, you can take the so-called "mini-pill" (an oral contraceptive containing progesterone only, rather than a combination of estrogen and progesterone), along with natural estrogen, until it is certain that menopause has arrived. If you are perimenopausal and are not taking HRT, you can use either the mini-pill alone or a low-dose combination contraceptive pill. The mini-pill will offer you a greater than 95-percent protection against pregnancy, and in many cases much better if ovulation is infrequent. A low-dose combination contraceptive pill will give you greater than 99-percent protection. If you are a smoker or have high blood pressure, it is safer to avoid all contraceptive pills containing estrogen, although the mini-pill, which contains progesterone only, can be used safely. Alternatively, physical methods of contraception—such as the diaphragm, cervical cap, intrauterine device (IUD), or condoms—can be used until menopause has definitely arrived.

Generally, doctors recommend that you use some form of contraception until you have had no menstrual periods for a year. After that, you should be able to relax and stop worrying about pregnancy. It is extremely unlikely you would conceive after more than a year without a menstrual period. Also, if you have an elevated blood level of follicle-stimulating hormone (over 30 milli-international units per milliliter; see page 8) that would indicate you are menopausal and therefore beyond your fertile stage.

The Vital Physical Examination

The physical portion of the examination should take about twenty minutes, and you'll be required to get into your birthday suit for the occasion. Your doctor will check your weight, pulse, and blood pressure; listen to your heart; and inspect your blood vessels, especially the veins in your legs. The thyroid gland, that soft, fleshy mound in the front of your Adam's apple, will be pressed, and your doctor should palpate (examine with his or her hands) your neck and armpits for any lumps or swelling. Your breasts should be thoroughly examined for any tenderness, lumpiness, or thickening. The skin and nipples of the breasts should also be inspected. Then your abdomen will be checked.

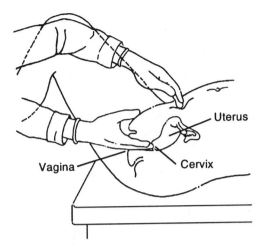

Figure 3.2 The Pelvic Examination

Finally, the doctor will do a pelvic examination (see Figure 3.2). The vagina and vulva should be checked for signs of estrogen deficiency or disease processes. The mucous membrane lining the vulva and vaginal wall will be checked, and an instrument called a speculum will be gently inserted to open up the vagina to expose the cervix. This allows a Pap smear to be taken (see Figure 3.3). This is a procedure in which the doctor scrapes cells from the cervix, using a spatula or a small brush. These cervical cells are then examined under a microscope for signs of changes that may signal developing cancer.In a woman with an estrogen deficiency, the vaginal secretions are scanty and alkaline (nonacidic), and the mucous membrane lining the vulva and vagina may be thin and fragile. Understandably, in such cases the taking of a Pap smear may be uncomfortable. It may be necessary to use a vaginal estrogen cream for one month to restore the vaginal tissues to normal so that a Pap smear and pelvic examination can be done comfortably.

You will be asked to cough or bear down while your doctor views the vaginal opening. This is done to reveal any tendency to prolapse of the uterus, bladder, and/or vagina, a situation that occurs when the ligaments and muscles supporting these organs weaken, causing them to fall downward and protrude through the vaginal opening. Next comes what I affectionately call the "squeeze test," as the doctor palpates with two hands your uterus, ovaries, and surrounding pelvic organs. This is a vital part of your checkup, as the only early evidence of cancer of the ovary is a swelling or lump in the pelvis. Try to relax

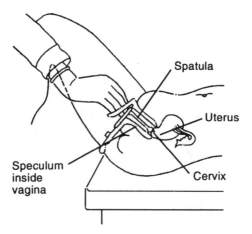

Speculum
inside
vagina

Spatula

Uterus

Cervix

Figure 3.3 Taking a Pap Smear

and breathe deeply during this procedure. It will make the pelvic examination more comfortable—and far more accurate. Making sure you have emptied your bladder before your examination is also a great help, especially when your doctor is squeezing around in your pelvis, checking the size and consistency of your uterus.

If your uterus is enlarged, or if your ovaries are enlarged or difficult to feel because you are overweight or tense, it is wise to have an ultrasound scan of your pelvis. This can reveal uterine fibroids (fibrous growths in the uterus) or tumors and cysts on the ovaries. Cancer of the ovaries becomes more common during the postmenopausal years and carries a very high risk of death, because it produces few symptoms in the early stages. Ovarian cancer is the fifth deadliest cancer in women and kills twice as many women as cancer of the cervix. It is usually discovered in women over the age of forty-five, at a stage when it has spread extensively. In general, it is a slow-growing cancer that is not diagnosed until late. An ultrasound scan can help to discover growths on the ovaries in the earlier and more curable stages. The more frequent use of ultrasound scans of the pelvis to check the ovaries in women over forty-five should reduce the currently pessimistic statistics for ovarian cancer.

Table 3.1 gives an overview of tests your doctor will probably perform during your physical examination and what he or she will be looking for.

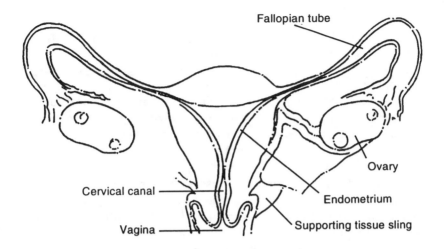

Figure 3.4   The Female Reproductive Tract (Front View)

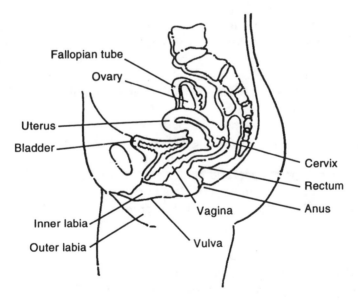

Figure 3.5   The Female Reproductive Tract (Side View)

Special Tests

Ideally, all women should begin to have biannual mammograms, or breast x-rays, at the age of forty years. The reason for this is that mammograms can detect breast cancer before a palpable lump has developed, and increase the rate of early detection. Early detection of breast cancer increases survival rates.

At the very least, you should have a mammogram at the time of menopause, if you are over forty, and especially before beginning HRT. This is because if you have a tiny, undiagnosed cancer lurking in your breast, HRT could stimulate its growth. Thus, it is important to rule out the presence of breast cancer before beginning HRT, and a mammogram is the most accurate means of doing this. Your doctor will examine your breasts very carefully for signs of cancer, but even the best doctor in the world can miss a tiny cancer because it is just too small to feel. A good-quality low-radiation-dose mammogram can reveal very tiny cancers, as small as one to two millimeters in size, long before you or your doctor would be able to feel it. In Sweden, studies have proven that routine screening of women aged forty-five years and over with regular mammograms can reduce deaths from breast cancer by up to 60 percent.

In addition to mammograms, a menopausal woman should have a bone mineral density test to measure the strength of her bones. This will enable your doctor to assess whether you are showing signs of osteoporosis and, if you are, to recommend treatment to try to rebuild bone, or at least to slow bone loss. Ideally, you should have a BMD test done when you reach menopause and at regular intervals thereafter (see page 27).

Other tests that should be performed include a complete blood count to check for anemia, as well as blood tests to check your liver function and measure your levels of follicle-stimulating hormone, estrogen, blood sugar, and cholesterol. If you have a past history of thrombosis (the formation of clots in the blood vessels), then blood should be taken for a clotting factor profile.

FOLLOW-UP VISITS

All postmenopausal women should see their doctors annually. If you are using only natural therapies, such as herbs and nutritional supplements, then the frequency of follow-up visits will vary, depending on your symptoms. However, an annual checkup should still be done. Using natural therapies is more of a self-help enterprise than HRT is. Unless you are working with a nutritionally oriented physician, you may prefer to visit your local health food store or a naturopathic physician for advice about adjusting your dosages of vitamins, for

Table 3.1 A Menopause Examination Checklist

This table provides you with a general checklist of important tests that are often performed at menopause, together with what the doctor is looking for when doing them. Your doctor will decide if any special tests, such as blood tests or pelvic ultrasound, are needed in your individual case.

Examination	What the Doctor Looks For
THE PHYSICAL EXAMINATION	
Heart, blood pressure, blood vessels	High or low blood pressure; signs of cardiovascular disease; varicose veins.
Weight	Underweight; obesity.
Thyroid gland	Enlargement; lumps. Under or over-activity can be confirmed with a blood test for thyroid function.
Breasts	Lumps; thickening; skin or nipple changes.
Abdomen	Swelling; tenderness.
Pelvic examination	Size of pelvic organs; condition of ovaries; signs of cancer, prolapse of uterus or bladder, vaginal atrophy.
SPECIAL TESTS	
Pap smear	Cancerous or precancerous cells in the cervix.
Mammogram	Very early signs of breast cancer.
Bone mineral density test (BMD)	Signs of osteoporosis.
Blood count; blood tests for estrogen, follicle-stimulating hormone (FSH), blood sugar, liver function, cholesterol level	Blood estrogen level; signs of metabolic disorders.
Urinalysis	Signs of infection, kidney disease.
Pelvic ultrasound	Signs of disease of the uterus and/or ovaries. Pelvic ultrasound is useful for women in whom pelvic examination is difficult, uncomfortable, or inconclusive.

example. You will also find Chapters 6 and 7, which discuss natural therapies and nutrition in detail, to be invaluable. The material in these chapters is based on my many years of clinical research into the use of herbs, vitamins, minerals, and essential fatty acids to relieve menopausal symptoms.

If you decide to try hormone replacement therapy, you will probably make this decision during your second visit to the doctor, at which time you and your doctor can review and discuss the results of all your tests. You may decide to start taking HRT immediately, or you may feel you need time to think about it, to seek a second opinion, or to sort out your feelings about HRT. The most pressing reason to begin estrogen replacement without delay would be a poor result on your bone mineral density test, which would mean that you are at high risk of developing osteoporosis.

If you decide to try HRT, monitor its effects by keeping a weekly record of your symptoms on your estrogen deficiency chart (see page 12). After you start HRT, your doctor will probably recommend follow-up appointments after two months, six months, and twelve months, and thereafter at twelve-month intervals. This will enable your doctor to fine-tune your HRT to suit your individual needs. A general physical examination, Pap smear, and mammogram should be repeated every twelve months. If the results of your initial bone mineral density test are satisfactory, this test can be repeated every three to five years. If the test shows a low mineral content in your bones, you should have additional bone mineral density tests done every one to two years.

If irregular, unexplained vaginal bleeding occurs twelve months or more after menopause, whether you are on HRT or not, a curettage of the uterus or a hysteroscopy should be done by a gynecologist. Some experts feel that all women on long-term HRT should have more than a Pap smear every twelve months. They recommend the addition of a test called an endometrial biopsy, in which a sample of cells from the lining of the uterus is taken and examined under a microscope. This is done to check for precancerous cells in the uterus, above the cervix. It can easily be done at the time of your annual Pap smear.

I hope that, after reading about all of the various aspects of your anatomy and biochemistry that require regular surveillance, you will be more inspired and less forgetful about making your visits to the doctor. I am horrified when I see a woman on HRT who has never had a breast examination or a mammogram, or a woman who believes, because she is using only natural therapies for menopause, that she no longer needs an annual Pap smear. I have also met older women who feel that their doctors are not interested in checking their breasts and genital organs, and who feel embarrassed to ask about it. This is sad—and also potentially dangerous. To safeguard your health in your menopausal and postmenopausal years, it is more important than ever before that you find a sympathetic doctor whom you can trust and with whom you can communicate.

Chapter 4

EVERYTHING YOU WILL EVER NEED TO KNOW ABOUT HORMONE REPLACEMENT THERAPY

Hormone replacement therapy is an option for every menopausal woman, but the decision to take it should be her own, based on accurate information and her individual lifestyle and health requirements. In addition, different HRT regimens are appropriate for different women. Some women need to take estrogen only; others require combination HRT, including both estrogen and progesterone. Hormones are often taken in tablet form, but some women fare better using other methods of administration, such as patches or injections.

In order to make an informed decision about taking HRT, you need to know about all the choices available to you, and their comparative advantages and disadvantages. In this chapter I will provide you with complete information about all the options available today, so that you will be able to make the decision that is right for you.

ESTROGEN

The basic element of any program of hormone replacement therapy is estrogen. This powerful sex hormone exerts effects throughout the body. Among other things, it helps to keep your skin soft, your bones strong, and your arteries clear.

Estrogen is available in different forms. One of the first and most important issues to understand, if you are considering hormone replacement therapy, is the distinction between natural and synthetic estrogen. There is a tremendous difference between the two.

Synthetic Estrogen

Synthetic estrogens are manufactured in laboratories. They are chemically foreign to the body's metabolic systems and so are not easily broken down by the body's natural enzymes. Consequently, they can accumulate in the body, causing them to exert stronger effects than the natural estrogens. Synthetic estrogens can also cause metabolic changes in the liver, leading to an increased incidence of side effects such as fluid retention, blood clots, aching legs, and high blood pressure. I prefer to avoid giving synthetic estrogens to menopausal and postmenopausal women. Natural estrogens are so much safer and are now widely available. In addition to ethinyl estradiol, which is marketed under various brand names, synthetic estrogens include quinestrol (sold under the brand name Estrovis) and diethylstilbestrol (better known as DES).

Natural Estrogen

Natural estrogen is mostly developed in laboratories, where an exact chemical replica of your ovaries' estrogen is cleverly synthesized. Although it may seem like a paradox to say that something natural can be synthesized, the important thing is that the end product is a hormone identical to the one produced by your own ovaries. Your body treats the synthesized natural estrogen exactly as it would your ovarian estrogen—it cannot tell any difference.

One popular type of natural estrogen, called Premarin, is extracted from the urine of pregnant mares. Premarin contains a mixture of natural humanlike estrogen (estrone sulfate) and some more potent equine (horse) estrogens. (So I suppose you could say that, strictly speaking, Premarin is natural only for horses!) In general, Premarin is an excellent form of replacement estrogen for menopausal women. However, because of its potency it can cause metabolic changes in the liver. For this reason, it should probably not be used by women who are obese, who smoke cigarettes, or who suffer from high blood pressure, high cholesterol, or varicose veins.

The most common truly natural estrogens are estropipate (sold under the brand name Ogen) and estradiol (Estrace and Estraderm). These natural estrogens are familiar to our bodies' metabolic systems and are easily broken down into forms that can readily be excreted by the liver and kidneys once they have been utilized and done their job. They do not accumulate in the body and are therefore less likely to cause side effects than the synthetic estrogens are. For these reasons, all women on HRT should be using the safer, natural estrogens.

Because natural estrogens are readily metabolized (broken down) by the body, if you take them in tablet form, you may need to take them twice daily (at twelve-hour intervals) to maintain adequate blood levels of estrogen at all times. It is not uncommon to see women on a once-a-day regimen of natural estrogen tablets who complain of hot flashes, vaginal dryness, fatigue, and other symptoms of estrogen deficiency. Blood tests often reveal that such women have inadequate levels of estrogen. In such cases, women usually experience great improvement if they take their estrogen tablets at twelve-hour rather than twenty-four-hour intervals.

Estrogens Most Often Used for HRT

Table 4.1 lists some of the estrogen tablets most commonly prescribed for HRT. As you can see, the daily dosages of estrogen tablets vary considerably in amount, depending on how rapidly your enzymes break them down, as well as on which brand of estrogen is prescribed. For example, estradiol is three times stronger than estropipate, and ethinyl estradiol is thirty times stronger than estradiol. In all cases, you must be guided by your own doctor in finding your required dose. Perimenopausal women (women in the years leading up to, during, and just after the final menstruation, roughly ages forty-five to fifty-five) still produce their own hormones erratically, and generally need higher doses of HRT than women in their late fifties or sixties.

PROGESTERONE—THE BALANCING HORMONE

In addition to estrogen, the ovary also makes the female sex hormone progesterone. Progesterone balances the effects of estrogen on the uterus and is necessary to produce regular periods.

If a woman with a uterus is taking replacement estrogen, it is now universally accepted that she must also take progesterone for at least ten to twelve days every calendar month in order to prevent uterine cancer. If estrogen is taken alone, there is an increased risk of cancer of the uterus. It is most reassuring to know that if a woman on HRT takes progesterone in addition to estrogen, her risk of uterine cancer actually *decreases*, to the point where it is lower than that of a woman who is not on HRT!

Table 4.1 Estrogen Tablets

This table lists some of the most common tablet forms of estrogen used in hormone replacement therapy. Note that dosages vary, depending both on the type of estrogen used and on the individual.

Product Name (Brand Names)	Type of Estrogen	Daily Dosage Range	Minimum Daily Dose Required to Prevent Osteoporosis
Chlorotrianisene (TACE)	Synthetic	12.0–25.0 mg	12.0 mg
Equine estrogen (Estratab, Premarin)	Natural	0.3–1.25 mg	0.625 mg
Equine estrogen plus testosterone (Estratest, Premarin with methyltestosterone)	Estrogen is natural; testosterone is of synthetic type	0.625–1.25 mg	0.625 mg
Estradiol (Emcyt, Estrace, Estraderm)	Natural micronized	1.0–4.0 mg	2.0 mg
Estropipate (Ogen)	Natural	0.625–2.5 mg	1.25 mg
Ethinyl estradiol (Brevicon, Demulen, Loestrin, and others)	Synthetic	0.01–0.03 mg	0.02 mg
Quinestrol (Estrovis)	Synthetic	0.01–0.02 mg	0.01 mg

Expert opinion is somewhat divided as to the necessity of adding some progesterone to estrogen replacement for a woman without a uterus (a woman who has undergone a hysterectomy). Some studies show that progesterone taken for twelve days every calendar month may exert a protective role against breast cancer, but this has not been categorically proven and debate on the subject continues. I personally would not recommend progesterone to a woman without a uterus.

Currently, the progesterone tablets that are commonly used along with estrogen in HRT contain synthetic progesterone. Synthetic forms of progesterone are called *progestogens*. Progestogens are not as good as natural progesterone, because they do not quite fit the progesterone receptors on your cells. However, they do still balance the effect of estrogen on the uterus.

Some of the progestogens currently used can have adverse effects on cholesterol levels, which may reduce the beneficial effect of estrogen on the blood vessels (see Table 4.2). While the debate continues, it is best to be guided by your doctor and use a progestogen such as Provera that will not cause ill effects on your cholesterol balance.

Some women refuse to take any progestogen tablets because they can cause such annoying side effects as irritability, depression, headaches, weight gain, bloating, and pelvic pain. If the side effects are intolerable, progestogen tablets can safely be omitted for a woman who has had a hysterectomy. If you have a uterus, you can discuss with your doctor the option of omitting progestogens. Another option for a woman who still has her uterus is to take natural progesterone injections every one to two days for twelve days out of every calendar month. In my experience, progesterone injections are very well tolerated and free of side effects, although because they are oily, some tenderness may be felt in the buttocks, the site of the injection. Progesterone injections act in a similar way to progestogen tablets in regulating the menstrual cycle and bringing on regular monthly bleeding. Natural progesterone has very few side effects and is better tolerated than the synthetic progestogens, which may cause side effects in susceptible women. In particular, natural progesterone does not cause the depression or unpleasant moods that progestogens sometimes do.

Natural progesterone is made from soybeans and yams. The required dosages are quite high, ranging from 200 to 400 milligrams daily for ten to twelve days out of every calendar month. These higher doses are necessary because natural progesterone is not as potent as the synthetic progestogens are. The main drawbacks of natural progesterone tablets, suppositories, and injections are that they are relatively expensive and some doctors are unfamiliar with their use. However, if you feel great while taking estrogen alone, only to find that once you add in the synthetic progestogen your mental and physical well-being deteriorate, then natural progesterone may hold the key to health and happiness for you. If your doctor is unfamiliar with natural progesterone products, you can encourage him or her to contact the Madison Pharmacy Association in Madison, Wisconsin, or O'Brien Pharmacy in Kansas City, Missouri, for more information. These companies sell pure natural

Table 4.2 Progesterones

This table lists some of the forms of progesterone that can be used in hormone replacement therapy. Note that dosages and method of administration vary, depending both on the type of progesterone used and on the needs of the individual.

Product Name (Brand Names)	Type of Progesterone	Daily Dosage Range	Advantages	Disadvantages
Medroxyprogesterone acetate (Amen, Curretab, Cycrin, Provera)	Synthetic	2.5–20 mg	Does not cause adverse effects on cholesterol.	May cause PMS-like symptoms.
Norgestrel (Ovrett)	Synthetic	0.03–0.09 mg	May reduce menstrual bleeding.	May exert masculinizing effects and increase weight and cholesterol levels.
Norethindrone (Aygestin, Micronor, Norlutate, Norlutin)	Synthetic	0.35–5 mg	May reduce breast tenderness.	May exert masculinizing effects, although not as much as norgestrel. May cause weight gain and increase cholesterol levels.
Progesterone tablets and suppositories	Natural	200–400 mg	No side effects, although suppositories may cause some vaginal irritation. No adverse effect on cholesterol.	Relatively expensive. Absorption may be less reliable.
Progesterone USP injections (progesterone in peanut or sesame oil)	Natural	100–500 mg	No side effects.	Injection site may become tender or inflamed.

micronized progesterone in a variety of forms, including tablets, capsules, suppositories, creams, and troches (small lozenges designed to dissolve when held against the inside of the cheek). *Micronized* progesterone is progesterone that has been broken into tiny particles so that it is better absorbed and utilized.

If you find you are unable to tolerate the side effects that progestogens or even natural progesterone may produce, you can ask your doctor's permission to leave them out completely, but if you do, you will have to have your endometrium (the lining of your uterus) checked every twelve months with a biopsy or hysteroscopy. As a last resort, if you feel very unwell without estrogen replacement, and yet feel even worse on progestogens, a hysterectomy could be a possibility. This is a drastic measure, but it is a possible option if you are very worried about increasing your risk of uterine cancer from unopposed estrogen replacement.

TESTOSTERONE

Janet, a fifty-six-year-old woman, was having a stressful menopause despite taking estrogen and progesterone tablets regularly. Her hot flashes and sweats made her feel dirty, her clothes clung to her flesh, and she felt as if ants were crawling under her skin. Her libido had vanished and a deep depression had set in. Janet had been told that these symptoms were all in her mind and that what she needed was a good psychiatrist. A blood test revealed low levels of estradiol and testosterone, so we decided she should take both estrogen and testosterone. Three weeks later, her blood test showed normal levels of estrogen and testosterone, and Janet was relieved of the symptoms that were supposedly "all in her mind."

Some of the psychological and sexual problems that can occur after menopause may be helped by taking the hormone testosterone. Generally, this is necessary only for a few months. Testosterone does not work as well when taken in tablet form, and an intramuscular injection of natural testosterone provides a better alternative.[1] Testosterone injections usually produce a feeling of mental, physical, and sexual well-being, and most women are very happy with the effects. However, it is only fair to warn any woman who is considering taking testosterone that it may cause a slight increase in facial hair or pimples (although this decreases when the dosage is reduced or the testosterone is discontinued). If the dose of testosterone is kept at 25 to 50 milligrams intramuscularly every three to six months, it is highly unlikely that undesirable

side effects such as facial hair, acne, voice changes, or increased cholesterol levels will occur. In some countries, testosterone is taken in the form
of hormonal implants, as well as by injection.

TAKING ORAL HRT

The most widely used and best known form of HRT is the oral, or
tablet, form, and most of the research on HRT has been done using
this form. Most women who take HRT are happy to take tablets of
estrogen and progesterone on a cyclical basis, in much the same
fashion that oral contraceptive pills are taken. Hormone tablets can
be taken according to many different time and dosage schedules.
Your doctor will work with you to determine the appropriate timing
and dosage for you, depending on your response to HRT and, to a
certain extent, on your lifestyle.

One of the most important points to understand about HRT is that if
you still have a uterus—that is, if you have not had a hysterectomy—you
must take progesterone in addition to estrogen for at least ten to twelve
days out of every calendar month. This will ensure regular monthly
bleeding and greatly reduce your risk of developing cancer of the uterus.
In fact, there is less of a risk of this type of cancer in women on
combination HRT than there is in women who take no hormone replacement at all. Estrogen tablets are often taken once or twice daily for
twenty-one or twenty-five days, with a five-day break between courses,
and with progesterone tablets being taken for the last twelve days of the
course (see Figures 4.1 and 4.2.). Menstrual bleeding usually occurs
during the five-day break from the estrogen tablets.

Can Menstrual Bleeding Be Avoided?

My catch phrase for the 1990s is "designer HRT." This refers to the fact
that today every woman who wants HRT can have it tailor-made to suit
her unique needs. A lot of older postmenopausal women stop HRT
because they don't want monthly menstrual bleeding. This is a pity, as
designer HRT can reduce or completely eliminate menstrual bleeding.

Some women feel better having a five-day break from estrogen, but
if you don't, there is no harm in taking estrogen every day. In fact,
taking estrogen every day is better for your bones and blood vessels.
There is no risk, provided you also take your progesterone tablets for
at least twelve days of each calendar month (see Figure 4.3).

Nowadays, older women are often prescribed both estrogen and

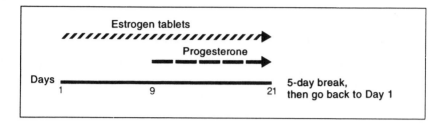

Figure 4.1 A Sample 21-Day HRT Cycle

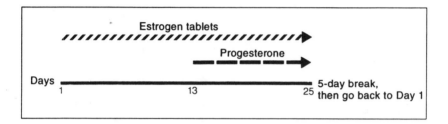

Figure 4.2 A Sample 25-Day HRT Cycle

progesterone tablets to be taken every day without a break, which completely eliminates menstrual bleeding. If any spotting or breakthrough bleeding occurs on this program, you may take a seven-day break from the estrogen and progesterone tablets every three months, which enables your uterus to shed any built-up lining in the form of a light menstrual period. Some women feel more comfortable having menstrual bleeding every three months or so, seeing it as a kind of "spring cleaning" for the uterus, after which they often feel better.

If you are a postmenopausal woman over the age of sixty-five and it is thought necessary for you to begin taking HRT for the first time to slow the progression of osteoporosis, you may take a small dose of estrogen continuously with no breaks at all. In such cases, light menstrual bleeding can be brought on only two or three times a year by the addition of a two-week course of progesterone tablets. This reduces the annoyance of regular monthly bleeding. A single HRT pill should soon be available that combines the two sex hormones estrogen and progesterone and that can be taken every day without a break, eliminating menstrual bleeding completely.

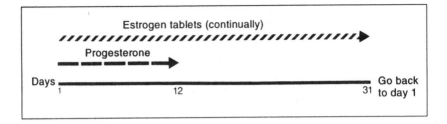

Figure 4.3 A Sample Monthly HRT Cycle With No Break Period

Every Woman Is Different

One woman's estrogen replacement needs may be two to four times higher than another's. Curiously enough, it is often the woman with a thin, lean build who needs greater amounts of estrogen. This is because such women tend to have very little production of estrogen from their fatty tissues. Furthermore, it is the thin, fine-boned woman who has a greater risk of osteoporosis and may need to take a greater amount of estrogen to prevent this.

Modern-day HRT has become so safe and effective in the prevention of many problems that every menopausal woman should be aware of its benefits. As long as no medical risks exist, HRT is an option about which you are entitled to make your own informed decision. However, it is true that menopausal women differ in their need for HRT. Some women say that they cannot live without it—they feel ancient, decrepit, and lifeless without estrogen in their bodies—while others hardly seem to notice when their ovaries finally stop producing estrogen. There are also some menopausal and post-menopausal women who actually feel worse on HRT, no matter what different forms and dosages are tried. Such was the story of Mandy, a big-boned, somewhat obese fifty-five-year-old woman who complained that she had gained over fifteen pounds and experienced fluid retention, aching legs, and fatigue since beginning HRT three years before. Her blood pressure was elevated and her legs were bulging with varicose veins. Mandy had started taking hormone tablets at the time of her natural menopause, without any blood tests or a bone mineral density check being done to assess her individual need for estrogen. I checked her bone mineral density and found it to be excellent. She had no risk factors for osteoporosis or heart disease.

In fact, her mother had lived to the age of ninety-eight with no trace of either osteoporosis or cardiovascular disease.

Thus, Mandy did not need to take HRT. Indeed, in her case, its side effects were greater than its benefits. She stopped HRT and six months later had lost thirteen pounds, regained her normal blood pressure, and generally felt much better. All Mandy needed was a doctor's permission to stop HRT, with the assurance that her bones and blood vessels would be checked regularly to make sure that she was not showing signs of developing osteoporosis or cardiovascular disease. In my opinion, Mandy was someone who did better without HRT. Menopausal women should not be made to feel that they must take HRT or else terrible things will happen to them. Rather, they should be given the information they need to make an informed decision. The merits of HRT vary for different individuals.

Hormone Replacement Therapy After Hysterectomy

More than half of American women have a hysterectomy by the age of sixty-five. HRT is simpler for women who have had a hysterectomy. In such cases, most experts agree that progestogen tablets are not necessary. An exception here is the woman who has a past history of endometriosis, a disorder in which cells from the endometrium (the lining of the uterus) are found growing outside the uterus, in the abdominal cavity. Endometriosis can be reactivated by estrogen replacement unless sufficient progesterone is taken to balance the estrogen therapy. Women with a past history of endometriosis (whether they have had a hysterectomy or not) should take low-dose progesterone tablets continually along with estrogen. If a woman has no past history of endometriosis, she can take estrogen by itself in the form of estrogen tablets, patches, or injections.

If the ovaries are conserved during hysterectomy in a woman not yet approaching menopause, they will usually function normally for many years after the operation. However, menopause may still arrive two to three years earlier than it would have otherwise. It is not uncommon for a woman to find that after hysterectomy, her ovaries do not work as well as they did before. She may complain of symptoms of estrogen deficiency. This is because the removal of the uterus can cause a reduction in the blood supply to the ovaries, and thus the ovaries no longer pump out adequate amounts of sex hormones. If this happens, a women can accurately be called premenopausal.

If you think this may be the case for you, compute your estrogen level score (see page 12), and if your score is around 20, ask your doctor for a blood test to measure levels of follicle-stimulating hormone, estrogen, and testosterone. If your FSH levels are elevated and your estrogen and testosterone levels are low, then your body is low in sex hormones. This may produce fatigue, depression, aches and pains, and loss of libido. A significant number of women in this situation find that hormone tablets do not alleviate these symptoms, and that they need to take either estrogen or estrogen and testosterone in non-tablet form, such as patches or injections. These may be better absorbed by the body than tablets are. If you try one of these types of HRT, you may find that your mental, physical, and sexual well-being soar to new heights, perhaps even better than before your hysterectomy.

If the ovaries are removed during hysterectomy, then the arrival of menopause is abrupt, and often severe symptoms of estrogen deficiency occur. This is particularly noticeable in younger women. Thankfully, estrogen replacement in the form of tablets, patches, or injections can stop unpleasant menopausal symptoms. If both ovaries are removed, a woman's testosterone level also may become very low (the ovaries produce testosterone as well as estrogen), so she may require testosterone replacement in the form of tablets or injections.

If you have had an endometrial ablation, you may still have some remnants of the uterine lining left behind and will need progesterone tablets to balance the effects of your estrogen replacement therapy on the endometrium. Endometrial ablation is a procedure in which high-frequency radio waves are used to ablate (destroy) the lining of the uterus, with the aim of reducing or stopping menstrual bleeding. (For a discussion of endometrial ablation, see Chapter 5).

NON-ORAL FORMS OF HRT

Although hormone tablets are the most commonly used type of HRT, they do not suit all menopausal women, either because of side effects or because of an inadequate response. It is important for you to be aware of other forms of hormone replacement that are not taken orally, such as patches, injections, and vaginal creams and suppositories. In many countries, hormones are also available as implants that are inserted into the fat of the buttocks or abdomen. These non-oral forms of hormone replacement are absorbed directly into the bloodstream, bypassing the digestive tract and the liver. This enables the hormones to travel directly to their target cells all over the body, where they exert their effects. After this they travel to the liver, where they are broken down and excreted.

Oral or tablet forms of hormones, on the other hand, must be absorbed from the intestines, and from there travel directly to the liver, where a significant amount of hormone is metabolized (broken down) before it passes into the circulation to travel to its target cells. The effect of hormones is thus weakened by this "first liver pass." Furthermore, large amounts of oral hormones passing through the liver tend to induce metabolic changes there, which may produce more side effects, such as fluid retention and elevated clotting factors in the blood.

If you are on hormone tablets and don't feel well, or find that your symptoms are not relieved, I suggest you ask your doctor about non-oral forms of hormones.

Hormone Injections

I first learned of estrogen injections when a remarkable New York journalist came to my office one day to get her "fix," as she called it—an estrogen injection. Melanie was a woman in her early sixties, but she looked at least twenty years younger. She related in her vivacious, extroverted way that she had been having one injection every month since her hysterectomy thirty years before. She was in excellent health, and her bone mineral density test did not reveal any signs of osteoporosis. This episode increased my interest in the usefulness of hormone injections, and I am eternally grateful for this to Melanie; hormone injections were not discussed at all in the curriculum at the medical school or at the teaching hospitals where I received my training.

Hormone injections were first manufactured and used in the 1930s and 1940s by German scientists and doctors. The injectable forms of hormones have proven to be popular among European women since the 1950s. They have been used only to a small degree by doctors in the United States. American doctors may be inexperienced with these injectable forms of HRT because they are not promoted at all by drug companies and clinical research material on their use is not widely available. Furthermore, some doctors feel that absorption from these injections is erratic, producing large fluctuations in the levels of hormones in the blood. Nevertheless, hormone injections continue to be popular in Europe.

I feel that there is a role for injectable forms of natural hormones.

Although I do not think they should be the first choice for all women, I have found that for some they can be more suitable than tablet forms. I myself am a migraine sufferer and cannot take tablet forms of estrogen. Indeed, estrogen tablets—both synthetic and natural forms—greatly aggravated my migraines, producing classic visual auras including flashing lights and blurred vision. After a hysterectomy for fibroids, I found that my ovaries became premenopausal and did not produce sufficient amounts of estrogen. I began receiving injections of natural estrogen into my buttocks every two weeks and found that for me, they really did the trick. They relieved my fatigue, loss of enthusiasm, aches and pains, and frequent headaches. My shrinking breasts became fuller, my libido returned, and my acne disappeared. I found that the injections produced a steady release of that wonderful hormone estrogen into my blood, provided I received them on a regular biweekly basis. To my relief, they were not painful. (Doctors are generally the biggest cowards and worst patients of all!) I did find that proper injection technique is most important; the needle should be placed deeply into the upper outer part of the buttock, which is the area with the greatest amount of fat. With this technique, the injection produces a slight dull stinging sensation lasting five to ten minutes, which is a small price to pay for the wonderful mental and physical well-being that the estrogen provides. Natural forms of the hormones estrogen, progesterone, and testosterone that are available in injection form are summarized in Table 4.3.

For some women (around 3 to 8 percent), the injections may be effective only temporarily. Such women find themselves requiring injections at increasingly shorter intervals, even through their blood tests show very high levels of estrogen. This is a type of addictive reaction called *tachyphylaxis*, in which it seems as if a woman simply cannot get enough estrogen. This is not good, as it is not natural for the body to continually have very high levels of estrogen, mainly because it theoretically increases the risk of breast or uterine cancer. Women who become "addicted" to high levels of estrogen should be switched to smaller dose estrogen patches. They can also benefit greatly from taking a number of nutritional and dietary supplements every day, including 3,000 milligrams of evening primrose oil, 50 milligrams of vitamin B_6, a balanced vitamin B complex, and antioxidants: 1,000 milligrams of vitamin C, 20 milligrams of beta-carotene, 500 international units of vitamin E, and 50 micrograms of selenium. This is because very high levels of estrogen may lead to nutritional deficiencies and imbalances in the body. A safe and reasonable level

Table 4.3 Injectable Natural Hormones

This table lists some of the forms of injectable natural hormones that can be used in hormone replacement therapy, together with the specific conditions for which they are generally recommended. Note that dosages and frequency of administration vary, depending both on the type of hormone used and on the needs of the individual.

Type of Hormone	Product Name (Brand Names)	Frequency of Injection	Conditions Used For
Estrogen	Estradiol cypionate (Depo-Estradiol)	One injection (5–10 mg) every two to four weeks.	• Menopause and premenopause; premature menopause; where other forms of estrogen replacement are ineffective. • Estrogen deficiency after hysterectomy or after surgical removal of the ovaries. • Some severe cases of premenstrual syndrome (PMS).
Estrogen and testosterone	Estradiol cypionate and testosterone cypionate (Depo-Testadiol)	One injection (100 mg testosterone and 4 mg estradiol) every four to twelve weeks. The prefix *Depo* denotes a storage injection that is long-acting, with effects lasting four to twelve weeks. Dosage can vary according to need. *Note:* Excessive doses of testosterone may cause acne, increased facial hair, and deepening of the voice. Best used on a temporary or intermittent basis.	• Difficult menopausal symptoms; hormonal deficiency after hysterectomy or removal of the ovaries. • Loss of libido, frigidity, poor sexual relationships. • Severe postnatal depression.
Progesterone	Progesterone USP injection	One injection (250–500 mg) every two or three days for ten to twelve days of every calendar month.	• Menopausal symptoms in women unable to tolerate oral progestogens. • Premenstrual syndrome (PMS). • Postnatal depression.

of estrogen in the body is around 82 to 136 picograms per milliliter (pg/ml), as determined by a blood test.

How Hormone Injections Transformed Two Women's Lives

Any doctor concerned with the well-being of menopausal women will realize that every woman is an individual and that it may be necessary to try different forms and dosages of HRT before physical and mental well-being can be restored. Miranda, age fifty-one, came to see me in a very distressed state. She had been on a standard dose of hormone tablets for two years but still complained of vaginal dryness and itching, poor libido, headaches, mood changes, insomnia, loss of confidence, and black depression. She was very frightened by these uncharacteristic changes in herself and felt she was becoming dependent on sedatives. Her psychiatrist—a man—told her that it could not be her hormones acting up, as she was on estrogen tablets. He told her she should give up working and concentrate more on her husband's needs. He also prescribed a large dose of antidepressant drugs and told her that she would need them to lead a normal life.

Miranda had scratched her vagina and vulva to the point that the area had developed fissures (dry cracks), and would often bleed after attempts at sexual intercourse. Her blood tests revealed lowish levels of estrogen, so I asked her to double her dose of estrogen tablets and use a vaginal estrogen cream. After three months on this increased dosage, she returned complaining that her migraines had worsened and that she had experienced only a slight improvement in the vaginal dryness and itching. Her fits of deep depression persisted and her marital situation had deteriorated. I then suggested that her liver was probably very active in breaking down the estrogen tablets, so that only small amounts of estrogen were getting past her liver to the rest of her body, which was still crying out for estrogen. We decided to try a course of natural estrogen and testosterone injections called Depo-Testadiol. This was injected every four weeks, and Miranda took a course of progesterone tablets for ten days out of every month to ensure that regular menstrual bleeding occurred.

One month after the first Depo-Testadiol injection, Miranda returned asking for another injection. She was delighted with the results of the first injection, which had given her a 90-percent improvement in all her symptoms. Her vagina had become moist and responsive, her libido was fantastic, her depression had lifted, and her husband was relieved to rediscover the girl he had married. She felt like socializing again and rejoining her exercise classes, and her mental efficiency at work had improved by leaps and bounds. Miranda received a course of three Depo-Testadiol injections, and then we decided she should continue taking natural estrogen in the form of hormonal patches (see page 67). That was several years ago, and she has never looked back. Her marriage is thriving, she has thrown out her sedatives and antidepressants, and she continues to enjoy her high-powered job. This is one of many success stories demonstrating that time, patience, and confidence in using the correct type of HRT for each individual woman will usually work.

Miranda was one of the significant percentage of women who do not find relief from estrogen deficiency symptoms with estrogen tablets. These women should not be told patronizingly that they have mental or emotional problems, or made to feel inadequate. Rather, they should be offered alternative forms of HRT such as injections or estrogen patches. If a doctor is not confident in this area, he or she should give an appropriate referral to another doctor or specialist with expertise in the field.

Another interesting story is that of forty-three-year-old Selina, who came to see me because of increasing premenstrual syndrome and a total loss of interest in sex. Selina craved more emotional and romantic attention from her fifty-eight-year-old husband, which he was unwilling to give because he resented her inability to satisfy his sexual appetite. They had been married when Selina was thirty-two, and things had been perfect until she underwent tubal ligation (surgical sterilization) at the age of thirty-five, after the birth of her second child. From that point on, Selina began to experience gradually increasing symptoms of estrogen and testosterone deficiency, including sudden mood changes, loss of sexual desire, and a reduction in the amount and frequency of her menstrual bleeding. A sample of Selina's blood revealed low estrogen and very low testosterone levels, consistent with a premenopausal state. To make matters worse, the amount of sex hormone binding globulin (SHBG) her liver was producing was very high. Sex hormone binding globulin is a protein in the blood that binds to and carries the sex hormones estrogen, progesterone, and testosterone in the bloodstream. Sex hormones are inactive when they are bound to sex hormone binding globulin, so the presence of large amounts of SHBG reduces the active role that sex hormones can play in your body. This was Selina's dilemma: low amounts of sex hormones and a high amount of sex hormone binding globulin circulating around in her body. She didn't stand a chance of feeling sexy, and things could only get worse as she got closer to menopause.

Selina and I designed a six-month program of estrogen and progesterone tablets for her, but she returned after four months, saying that her premenstrual irritability and sexual disinterest persisted. We then began a six-month course of monthly natural hormone injections. Selina received an injection of Depo-Testadiol (estrogen and testosterone) at the end of every menstrual period, and one Depo-Estradiol (estrogen) and one progesterone injection on the sixteenth day of every menstrual cycle. This produced a dramatic improvement in her mental, physical, and sexual well-being. Her husband could hardly keep up with this newly energetic and sexual woman. The combination of these three injections, containing natural estrogen, testosterone, and progesterone, had provided Selina's brain, genital organs, and other sexually responsive body cells with sex hormones that her own premenopausal ovaries could not provide. After six months, Selina found a slight increase in facial hair, so we stopped the Depo-Testadiol injections, which contain testosterone. She eventually opted for an implant of natural estrogen without any testosterone, as her libido had returned to normal and she did not want any increase in facial hair.

Selina's case illustrates one of the many flexible programs of "designer HRT" that can be tried for women with hormonal imbalances in the premenopausal years. The injectable forms of natural hormones are very useful for what I call a "hormonal crisis," a severe and/or sudden deficiency or imbalance in hormones such as may occur after a hysterectomy, surgical removal of the ovaries, tubal ligation, sudden onset of menopause, premature menopause, a severe medical illness, severe stress, chemotherapy treatment for cancer, or childbirth. Natural hormone injections can truly work wonders, and can prevent a hormonal crisis from leading you into a deep, dark pit; indeed, they usually take you out of the pit quickly and efficiently. Depending on the cause of your problem, you may need them for only three to six months, until your own hormones recover, or you may continue to need estrogen and find it more convenient to take estrogen tablets or use estrogen patches.

Estrogen Patches

Who would ever have thought that one day we would come up with the idea of applying sticky Band-Aids containing estrogen to our skin to help us remain well and feminine? The idea is here to stay, and women in America, Britain, and Switzerland have been using the patch for five to ten years now.

The natural estrogen in the patch is absorbed through the skin into the bloodstream. One patch can be worn for three days on a convenient part of the buttocks or torso (other than the breasts). The site selected should be one where little wrinkling of the skin occurs during movement of the body, such as the abdomen, buttock, or lower back. There is no need to take a break from using the patches. A woman with a uterus should take progesterone tablets also for ten to twelve days every month. Hopefully, in the near future we will have patches containing natural progesterone that can be used along with the natural estrogen patches.

Estrogen patches contain the natural estrogen estradiol, and are sold under the brand name Estraderm. They come in two different strengths: Estraderm 0.1 and Estraderm 0.05. Occasionally, the patches can produce local skin irritation and redness because they contain alcohol. To reduce this irritation, after peeling off the patch's adhesive cover, leave the sticky side of the patch exposed to the air for thirty minutes before applying it to your skin. This simple trick will often make a big difference. It helps to change the site of the patch with each successive application, and you can also use a vitamin E or cortisone cream on irritated skin after removing the patch. In a small number of women, the patch produces severe skin irritation and allergy, which necessitates changing to another form of HRT.

When the estrogen patch first appeared on the scene, there was some skepticism about its ability to be well absorbed into the bloodstream. However, the patches have undergone extensive testing and have been shown to produce very adequate blood levels of estradiol—indeed, levels similar to those found in younger women not yet approaching menopause, who still have natural menstrual cycles. A recent study reported in the British medical journal *Lancet* produced very exciting news about the ability of the estrogen patch to reduce calcium loss from the spinal vertebrae and hipbones. The 0.05 estrogen patch, which contains 4 milligrams of estradiol, was found to be just as effective as tablet forms of estrogen in the prevention of osteoporosis.[2] The estrogen patch is a very safe way for you to achieve constant and normal levels of estrogen in your blood. Because the estrogen is absorbed through the skin and directly into the bloodstream instead of through the digestive tract, it is able to reach your cells before it is broken down by the liver. Thus, smaller doses of estrogen can be used and side effects due to metabolic changes in the liver are far less likely. This makes the patch excellent for women with high blood pressure, fluid retention, bloating, varicose veins, obesity, and a past history of clots or thrombosis.

Take the case of Alice, a sixty-two-year-old woman who had been told that she could never take estrogen because she had suffered two serious blood clots in her leg, one after her hysterectomy at the age of forty-three and the other after an appendectomy at the age of forty-nine. Alice was following in her mother's footsteps as far as osteoporosis was concerned, and by the age of fifty-eight had developed an obvious hump on her back. X-rays revealed several crushed spinal vertebrae in her back, and her bone density values were very low and getting worse every year. Alice knew she needed estrogen, but she was afraid to take it because she feared that it would cause a recurrence of her blood clots. I persuaded Alice to try the estrogen patch and she began using it regularly. She was greatly relieved to be able to take a form of estrogen that was safe and effective, and we both relaxed six months later, when tests showed that she had stopped losing calcium from her spine.

The estrogen patch can be a godsend to women unable to tolerate estrogen tablets. It is also better for high-risk women, such as those with liver disorders, high blood pressure, varicose veins, or a history of thrombosis, and for those who cannot stop smoking. The patch is useful as well for women with bowel problems, such as Crohn's disease, ulcerative colitis, irritable bowel syndrome, and poor intestinal absorption, as these conditions may cause hormone tablets to be poorly absorbed.

Vaginal Estrogen

Estrogen can also be taken via the vagina. Indeed, this is a very popular form of HRT. It is particularly useful if you have a lot of vaginal dryness or shrinkage; it will also reduce bladder problems such as urinary frequency, incontinence, or a burning sensation with urination. Estrogen cream is easily inserted with a vaginal applicator, which enables you to place the cream high into the vagina. It is best done last thing at night before going to bed, after sexual intercourse, and after emptying the bladder. Estrogen is rapidly absorbed through the vaginal lining into the bloodstream, and reasonable levels of blood estrogens can be achieved.

Generally, vaginal estrogen cream is prescribed for once-a-week use, but you may use it more often if you desire. If you still have your uterus, the regular, frequent use of vaginal estrogen should be accompanied by a twelve-day course of progesterone tablets every two or three months to guard against estrogenic overstimulation of the uterus. These progesterone tablets may bring on a light menstrual period.

Some women find the vaginal estrogens are satisfactory and do not take any other forms of estrogen. Several women have told me that they feel very sexy several hours after using these creams! Others find the creams a little messy and prefer to use vaginal estrogen suppositories, which are inserted high into the vagina with an applicator. Regular estrogen tablets can also be inserted into the vagina. If they are placed high enough in the vagina, they are well absorbed. If you find that taking estrogen tablets orally is causing side effects such as nausea or fluid retention, you may find that changing to the vaginal route of administration will eliminate these side effects.

Hormone Implants

Hormone implants are small, solid pellets of natural hormones that resemble tiny pieces of spaghetti. They are implanted (inserted) into the fatty layer under the skin of the abdomen or buttocks. A doctor uses a local anesthetic and a small hollow tube with a sharp cutting edge to slide the pellet neatly into the fatty tissue. This procedure should not be painful. The implants release hormones slowly and directly into the bloodstream for six to twelve months, depending on the dosage.

Implants of natural estrogen and testosterone have been used for many years in Europe, South Africa, and Australia, where they are becoming increasingly popular. Unfortunately for American women, these hormone implants have not yet been approved by the U.S. Food and Drug Administration and are therefore not generally available in the United States. There are a few American doctors known to be working with hormonal implants, however, and it may also be possible for your doctor to import hormonal implants for you from overseas, provided he or she first applies to the FDA for permission to use the implants under an investigational exemption. However, hormone implants should be inserted only by doctors who have special expertise in this area. This is because if they produce unwanted side effects, removal of the implants can be difficult.

I believe that American women, including American doctors,

should lobby the FDA to study and approve the use of hormone implants. Their absence in America creates a gap in the range of hormonal products available for menopausal women. Of all the types of HRT, an implant comes closest to copying the function of your own ovaries, as in both cases estrogen is released directly into the bloodstream and is carried to the various estrogen-dependent tissues of your body. Implants are particularly good for menopausal women with severe symptoms and/or symptoms that do not respond to other treatment. It is definitely true that for a small percentage of women, no other type of HRT works as well as hormone implants. I have found this to be more likely in the following cases: after hysterectomy (surgical removal of the uterus); after oophorectomy (surgical removal of the ovaries), especially in younger women; and in premature menopause. Thus, I believe that even though hormone implants are not currently approved for sale in the United States, all menopausal women should know of their role and benefits.

As you can see, there are many different ways you can take hormone replacement. What works for one woman does not necessarily work for another, and time and patience may be needed to find out the correct dosages and form of HRT for you. I call this designer HRT, meaning that a particular regime of HRT can be tailor-made to keep you feeling well and to stabilize your blood levels of hormones in the normal range.

Chapter 5

The Most-Asked Questions About Menopause

Many women are confused about important aspects of menopause, and find it difficult to get direct and clear answers. When it comes to menopause, ignorance is *not* bliss. It can be frightening to feel that your body is going through incomprehensible changes over which you have no control.

Each section in this chapter is devoted to one of the questions my women patients ask me most often. It is designed to give you accurate answers and vital information that will enable you to make informed decisions. It will help to demystify menopause and put you back in control of your life and your health.

WHEN WILL I GO THROUGH MENOPAUSE?

The average age at menopause is fifty years. However, some women go through a premature menopause in their twenties or thirties, while others continue to menstruate until their late fifties.

There are a number of factors that are known to influence the age at which a woman experiences menopause. If you started menstruating early in life (before ten years of age), you are more likely to have a late menopause. On the other hand, if you have had a hysterectomy, even if you kept your ovaries, you may experience menopause up to four years earlier than average. This is because the blood supply to the ovaries may be decreased after removal of the uterus. Other factors associated with early menopause include smoking, radiation exposure, and chemotherapy. Menopause can also be brought on artificially if the ovaries are removed through surgery or if they are treated with radiation therapy.

HOW LONG DOES MENOPAUSE LAST?

The word *menopause* means the cessation of menstrual bleeding—that is, the last menstrual period. However, in the several years before, during, and after the last period, huge hormonal changes, such as large and sometimes rapid fluctuations in the levels of sex hormones, take place in the body. This period of time is called the *perimenopause* or the *climacteric*. Common symptoms are hot flashes, sweating, changes in menstrual bleeding, and mood changes. These symptoms may last for a variable period of time, and the variation among individual women is quite amazing. Some women find that perimenopause lasts only a few months, while others find that it lasts for ten to fifteen years. Thankfully, with appropriate HRT and/or natural therapies, you can avoid the unpleasant symptoms of this time altogether!

After the perimenopausal period, a woman becomes post-menopausal, with very low and stable levels of sex hormones in her body (unless, of course, she is taking hormone replacement therapy).

SHOULD I TAKE HORMONES?

When you look at the advantages and powerful influences of hormone replacement therapy, it is tempting to believe that all women should take estrogen for menopause. It can effectively relieve acute menopausal discomforts, such as hot flashes and flagging libido, and also dramatically reduces the risk of osteoporosis and cardiovascular disease. But each woman is unique. Some women have no symptoms and are not at risk of developing cardiovascular disease or osteoporosis, so there is no medical reason for them to take HRT. But every menopausal woman has the right to be examined and tested. And if you are found to be at risk of developing one of these serious health problems, or if you are suffering from unpleasant menopausal symptoms, you should be offered the option of taking HRT. Furthermore, there are many popular misconceptions about HRT (for a look at some of the more common ones, see Hormonal Myths on page 73). Consequently, all women should receive complete and accurate information about HRT before deciding whether or not to try it.

IF I TAKE HRT, HOW LONG WILL I NEED IT?

Around 40 percent of women still complain of symptoms due to estrogen deficiency ten years after the start of menopause. They may still be troubled by hot flashes, vaginal dryness, sweating, and loss of

Hormonal Myths

Many women are reluctant to consider hormone replacement therapy because of some of the things they may have heard about it. But many of these things are really nothing more than hormonal myths. The following table lists some of these common misconceptions as well as the actual facts about HRT.

Myth	Truth
If I start on HRT, I'll never be able to come off it.	Not true. HRT is not addictive.
Menopausal problems can always be fully treated with nutritional medicine.	Each woman is an individual. Some require estrogen replacement therapy for optimum health and well-being.
HRT should always be taken in the lowest possible dose for the shortest possible time.	Dosage needs vary with the individual. Some women should take HRT for at least fifteen to twenty years.
HRT never causes weight gain.	HRT can cause weight gain in some women, even if they do not eat more or exercise less (see page 75).
HRT increases the risk of cancer.	Properly balanced natural HRT actually reduces the risk of endometrial and ovarian cancer. In some cases it may increase the risk of breast cancer, although further long-term studies are required to demonstrate this. It appears to have little or no effect on other types of cancer.
If HRT brings back my periods, I might get pregnant.	This is impossible. A menopausal woman has no eggs left in her ovaries and without eggs, conception cannot occur.
I will not need HRT until after my menstrual bleeding ceases.	Not necessarily. A deficiency of estrogen may occur several years before this.
Menopause is a short-lived condition.	Menopause is an epoch with effects lasting until the end of life.

sexual desire and enjoyment. Such symptoms last for different periods of time in different people, so the appropriate duration of estrogen replacement therapy for the control of acute menopausal symptoms varies, depending on what an individual woman needs.

To prevent osteoporosis, estrogen replacement therapy must be taken for a period of fifteen to twenty years. Taking estrogen protects your bones against calcium loss and your heart and blood vessels against disease, but this protection ceases once estrogen therapy is stopped. Many doctors therefore believe that women at risk of developing osteoporosis should stay on estrogen for life, provided they feel well and receive regular medical checkups. Furthermore, it is never too late to begin HRT. Some women can still benefit if they start it in their sixties or seventies.

We know that fewer than one third of postmenopausal women continue with HRT over the long term. This is because many women feel uncomfortable about making a long-term commitment to HRT, as there is continuing controversy as to whether it may cause an increased risk of breast cancer or liver disease. I believe that the duration of HRT is a very individual matter that needs to be reviewed regularly throughout the postmenopausal period. Ultimately, the length of time you take HRT should be your informed choice. You will need to read all of this book and communicate with your doctor before you decide what is right for you.

WHAT IF I GET SIDE EFFECTS?

Usually, side effects from HRT are minor and can be overcome by trying smaller doses of hormones or taking a different form of HRT. Rarely, high doses of the oral forms of HRT can cause thrombosis (the formation of a blood clot or clots in the blood vessels), and this may produce pain and swelling in the legs. HRT may cause migraine headaches in women who are predisposed to them, and the migraines can be preceded by disturbances in vision or speech or by a sensation of weakness in the limbs. This is not common, but if it occurs you should immediately cease taking HRT and consult your doctor. Women more prone to such side effects are those who smoke, who are obese, or who have high blood pressure, varicose veins, or a past history of blood clots or strokes. For such high-risk women, estrogen patches are much safer than other forms of HRT.

Some women on HRT complain of a mild to moderate weight gain. This is because HRT may cause a slight increase in appetite and fluid retention. Weight gain can be avoided by reducing the dose of HRT, avoiding strong androgenic (masculinizing) progestogens such as norgestrel and norethindrone, reducing the amount of saturated fat in the diet, and getting regular exercise.

Fewer than 50 percent of women who start on HRT continue with treatment for more than a few months. Yet to prevent osteoporosis, HRT must be taken for fifteen to twenty years, if not for life. The reason many women give up on HRT is that they get annoying side effects. I have designed a table to help you and your doctor work out some practical solutions and alternatives if you run into problems with HRT (see Table 5.1). Remember, patience is a virtue!

Side effects can be minimized by starting with small doses of natural hormones and, if necessary, gradually increasing the dose until you feel relieved of your symptoms. Your doctor may need to adjust your dosage and method of taking HRT several times to find a program that suits you as an individual and avoids annoying side effects.

WON'T HRT MAKE ME GAIN WEIGHT?

In my experience, approximately one in three women who start hormone replacement therapy at menopause gains a significant amount of weight. This is usually in the range of four to five pounds, but it can occasionally be much more. This tendency can be avoided by asking your doctor to prescribe natural forms of estrogen and progesterone instead of the synthetic types of these hormones. Quite a few menopausal women find that they need to reduce the dosage of hormone replacement therapy or, if that fails, to take HRT in the form of estrogen patches instead of tablets to avoid gaining weight.

Estrogen patches are sold under the brand name Estraderm and come in two strengths: Estraderm 0.1 and Estraderm 0.05. The smaller dose of estrogen in the weaker estrogen patch—Estraderm 0.05—is most unlikely to cause weight gain. Generally speaking, it is possible, by juggling and/or reducing the doses of estrogen and progesterone in your hormone replacement therapy, to avoid any significant weight gain.

Heavier women usually require smaller doses of hormones than thin women do. They may need to take smaller amounts of progesterone, either by breaking the tablets in half or quarters, or by taking them for a shorter time each calendar month. Natural progesterone tablets are unlikely to cause any big gains in weight and may be preferred by women with weight problems.

If, despite all these measures, hormone replacement therapy still

Table 5.1 Problem Side Effects of HRT and Suggested Solutions

Many women who try hormone replacement therapy discontinue it because they are bothered by side effects such as weight gain, headaches, or fluid retention. Yet in many cases, side effects can be minimized or even eliminated by making adjustments in dosage or method of administration. The table below lists some of the most commonly cited troublesome side effects of HRT and suggested solutions for them. However, you should never make any changes in your HRT program without first consulting your doctor.

Side Effect	Suggested Solution
Breast swelling and tenderness, heavy menstrual bleeding, menstrual cramps.	Breast tenderness and heavy menstrual bleeding can be caused by too much estrogen. Reduce the dosage of estrogen and possibly increase the dosage of progestogen. Take 3,000 mg of evening primrose oil and 50 mg of vitamin B_6 daily.
Increased blood pressure, fluid retention, bloating, weight gain, aching legs.	Fluid retention can be caused by too much estrogen. Reduce the dosage of estrogen or change to a non-oral form such as patches. Reduce the dosage of progestogen.
Migraine headaches, nausea, vomiting.	Nausea and headaches can be caused by too much estrogen. Change to a non-oral form of estrogen such as patches. Begin with low-dose estrogen patches.
Inability to tolerate menstrual bleeding.	Take both estrogen and progestogen continuously, every day. Or consider endometrial ablation (see page 80).
Depression, irritability, mood changes, loss of sex drive.	Change to a non-oral form of estrogen such as patches or injections. The addition of testosterone injections may be necessary, often for three to twelve months only. Change to a natural progesterone.
Chloasma (dark and/or blotchy brown facial pigmentation).	Reduce the dosage of estrogen and change to estrogen patches. Avoid exposure to sunlight; wear a hat and sun block when outdoors.

Side Effect	Suggested Solution
Premenstrual symptoms such as depression and/or irritability during progestogen therapy.	Depression and symptoms of premenstrual syndrome can be caused by too much progestogen. Reduce the dosage of progestogen (to 2.5 mg of Provera daily, for example), or change to natural progesterone tablets, suppositories, or injections. Natural progesterone is less likely to cause mood disorders than synthetic progestogens are. Take progesterone less often, every two or three months instead of every month. Take 50 mg of vitamin B6 and 3,000 mg of evening primrose oil daily.
Estrogen deficiency symptoms while on HRT.	See the Estrogen Level Score Chart on page 12. Have a blood test to check your blood level of estradiol. If it is on the low side, increase the dosage of oral estrogen or add or change to estrogen patches or injections. For vaginal dryness, add estrogen cream.
Development of large varicose veins or worsening of existing varicose veins.	Reduce the dosage of estrogen or change to estrogen patches. Take 500 IU of vitamin E daily.

causes unwanted weight gain, you may decide to give up on HRT altogether, but check with your doctor first. You may be losing the great advantages that estrogen replacement therapy offers your skeleton and blood vessels. You may also benefit from specific changes in diet tailored to your individual metabolism (see Body Types and HRT on page 78).

If after all consideration you do decide to give up on hormone replacement therapy, I suggest that you consume plenty of foods that are high in calcium, vitamin D, and natural plant estrogens. Natural plant estrogens can be found in many foods, such as green beans and soybeans. Further information about foods that are high in natural plant estrogens and calcium may be found in Chapter 6.

IS THERE ANY WAY TO AVOID BLEEDING ON HRT?

Some postmenopausal women cannot cope with any bleeding, even if it is regular and predictable, at an age in life when they wish to be

Body Types and HRT

Weight gain is a not uncommon side effect of hormone replacement therapy. However, the exact way in which you may be affected depends on your body type. Generally speaking, all women fall into four different body type categories—android, gynecoid, lymphatic, and thyroid. You can be a combination of two of these four different types, but most women are predominantly one type or another.

The android type is characterized by a strong, sometimes thickset, skeletal frame, broad shoulders, a wide rib cage, and muscular limbs. The waist is not well defined and the pelvic bones are narrow, so that the physique is relatively straight up and down. There is a lack of feminine curves and the figure is somewhat "boyish." The buttocks and thighs are muscular and the pelvis and buttocks do not curve outwards below a somewhat thick waist. The android-type woman's limb bones are large, and she has more muscle mass and less fat tissue than the other body types. If excess weight gain occurs, fat is deposited in the upper part of the body, above the pelvis. This results in a thickening of the neck, torso, waist, and abdomen—the pattern sometimes called "apple-shaped obesity." An android-type woman, if taking excessive or unnecessary HRT, will put on weight in the upper portion of her body, especially if she is taking excessive progesterone or testosterone.

The gynecoid type is characterized by a pear shape, with the buttocks and thighs flowing outwards below a narrow waist. The buttocks are curved and rounded, and the thighs curve out to the sides. The shoulders are small to average in breadth; the waist is tapered and much smaller than the hips; and the pelvis is wide. The bones of the limbs are slender, with tapered, fine forearms, wrists, shins, and ankles. If weight gain occurs, fat is deposited first on the buttocks, thighs, and breasts, and later over the lower abdomen in front of the pubic bones, while the forearms and shins remain relatively slim. The bottom has a tendency to droop downward over the backs of the thighs if weight gain occurs. A gynecoid-type woman who takes excessive or unnecessary HRT will put on weight primarily in the pelvic area, buttocks, and thighs. This type of woman becomes more pear-shaped as she gains weight.

The lymphatic type is characterized by a generalized thickening and puffiness of the tissues underlying the skin. This is because she retains lymphatic fluid and fat, especially in her limbs, which gives her thick arms and legs, with a straight up and down look along their length. The ankles and wrists are thick and puffy in appearance. The shoulders, breasts, and rib cage are average in size, and the abdomen may protrude in front. The torso, like the limbs, is relatively straight up and down, with a thick waist and moderate curves outward on the buttocks and thighs. The bones and the muscles are average in size and their shape is not clearly defined. If a lymphatic-type woman gains excessive weight, the extra fat will be distributed all over her body—in the legs, feet, arms, hands, buttocks, abdomen, trunk, neck, and face. Lymphatic-type women gain weight very easily and often have been chubby since childhood. If a lymphatic-type woman takes excessive or unnecessary HRT, she will put on weight all over, in the form of an extra layer of fat over her entire body. She will also retain fluid in her limbs.

The thyroid type is characterized by a narrow streamlined shape, with fine bones and long limbs. Many thyroid-type women are tall, but even those who are not give the impression of being taller than they are, because of their relatively long legs and arms. They have narrow waists and small curves outwards on the buttocks and thighs. Their fingers, toes, and necks are long and narrow, like their limbs. Their bones are fine and the bone structure is clearly defined, with the ribs and bony protuberances (knobs) around the joints being very evident. If weight gain occurs, fat is deposited around the abdomen and upper thighs, while the upper part of the body and limbs remain slim. Thyroid-type women gain weight less easily than the other body shapes. Generally speaking, the thin thyroid types tolerate higher doses of HRT without significant weight gain.

If you have worked with your doctor to find the correct dose of HRT and you still find yourself gaining weight and don't know why, investigate your diet more thoroughly. You may be consuming excess calories or a diet that is wrong for your particular body shape. In my experience, each of the four body shapes has a different metabolism and hormonal balance, and you will lose weight most effectively if you follow a scientifically balanced diet and eat combinations of food that are right for your body shape. This unique weight-loss approach is called the Body Shaping Diet. A full discussion of this approach is available in my book, The Body Shaping Diet Book, which gives step-by-step meal plans and recipes formulated for each of the four body shapes to achieve effective weight loss and body shaping.[1]

free of periods, tampons, and inconvenient napkins and pads. If you feel like this, tell your doctor. He or she can prescribe progestogen tablets to be taken every day along with your estrogen therapy. This will usually prevent any bleeding after three to four months of continual therapy.

Some women prefer to work with their doctors to try to manipulate the doses of HRT to reduce the amount and/or frequency of bleeding. This can be done by taking the progestogen course once every two or three months, instead of monthly; by increasing the strength of the progestogen tablet; or by reducing the amount of estrogen.

A new surgical technique is now available that enables a surgeon to remove the endometrium (the lining of the uterus) while leaving the uterine walls intact. This is called *endometrial ablation*. In this procedure, the surgeon destroys the bleeding surface of the uterus with high-frequency radio waves or laser beams. Endometrial ablation can be done using a hysteroscope inserted through the cervix, so that no incision or stitches are required. This reduces the amount of pain, postoperative discomfort, and time off work the procedure entails. Since it is performed under general anesthesia, endometrial ablation is a hospital procedure, but it is usually considered outpatient surgery (no overnight hospital stay is required).

The success of endometrial ablation varies. Afterwards, you may find that you have no further bleeding or that the amount of bleeding is reduced to some degree. The amount of this reduction varies from woman to woman. For the best results, go to a gynecologist who has a lot of experience in performing hysteroscopy and endometrial ablation. After an endometrial ablation, it is still necessary to take some progesterone tablets every month (because you still have your uterus), but your menstrual bleeding will be much less or even nonexistent.

Some women become so annoyed and fatigued by the bleeding HRT produces that they consider the option of hysterectomy. This is because a woman without a uterus can take estrogen by itself without any progestogen and have no bleeding at all. A hysterectomy, however, is major surgery, and should be considered only when other measures, such as changes in the HRT regimen or endometrial ablation, offer no relief.

ARE THERE ANY REASONS I SHOULDN'T TAKE ESTROGEN?

Modern-day natural HRT is very flexible and safe, and only a minority of women are told by their doctors that they should avoid it.

However, if you suffer from or have a history of any of the following problems, you will probably be advised never to take estrogen:

• Estrogen-sensitive cancer, such as breast or endometrial cancer. Doctors generally are reluctant to give estrogen to women who have previously been treated for uterine cancer, because it is possible that estrogen may stimulate the distant spread of the cancer. However, if the cancer was detected in the early stages and was determined to be of a less aggressive type, and if the patient has remained cancer-free for at least two years, some doctors feel it is safe to prescribe estrogen in small doses if a patient complains of severe symptoms of estrogen deficiency. Some women who have been successfully treated for breast cancer find that they are unable to tolerate a complete lack of sex hormones in their bodies, and HRT programs using very small doses of estrogen and larger doses of progesterone can often be worked out for them. They may choose to take this type of HRT after weighing all the pros and cons with a cancer specialist. If the cancer has been completely removed and there is no sign of invasion into the local blood vessels, and the lymph glands in the armpits are free of cancer, there is roughly a 75-percent chance of a complete cure, and as far as we know, taking HRT does not dramatically change this. A woman may live another twenty to thirty years after successful treatment for breast cancer, and she may not want to run the increased risk of bone fracture or heart attack that can occur without estrogen.

• Severe liver disease, such as cirrhosis. Severe liver disease makes it difficult for your liver to break down or metabolize estrogen. Normal doses of estrogen replacement usually overtax a diseased liver so that liver function may worsen. Mild to moderate liver disease is not necessarily a contraindication to estrogen replacement, although in such a case I would advise that you use only estrogen patches or vaginal estrogen, as these are most unlikely to overtax your liver. It is best to avoid oral estrogens in all cases of liver disease. If you have liver disease, you will need to ask your gastroenterologist about the type of liver disease you have. Liver function is easily checked with a blood test.

There are several other medical problems that make many doctors very cautious about prescribing estrogen. They are not, however, absolute reasons that you cannot take HRT; you can, but extra vigilance and care is required. These medical problems are:

• Recent or severe blood clots or thrombosis. The statistical risk of blood clots is not increased by HRT, but if there is a past history of clots, many doctors prefer to use the estrogen patches, as they are the safest way of taking HRT.

• Mild liver disease (see page 81).

• Severe high blood pressure that is difficult to control with drugs.

• Fibroids or endometriosis. With HRT, pain and irregular bleeding can be a problem and surgical treatment may be required.

• Gallbladder disease. Gallbladder problems may be aggravated by HRT.

• Benign breast disease (mastopathy, fibrocystic disease of the breast, or chronic cystic mastitis). This may be aggravated by HRT.

• Systemic lupus erythematosus. Lupus may be aggravated by HRT.

If you are suffering from symptoms of estrogen deficiency but feel that estrogen replacement therapy is too dangerous for you, I recommend that you increase the amount of foods in your diet that are sources of natural plant estrogens (see Chapter 6).

WILL HRT INCREASE MY RISK OF CANCER?

If all the published literature and clinical trials to date are analyzed, it can be concluded that, generally speaking, death rates from all cancers are not increased by the correct use of HRT. However, very long term studies are not yet available. It will be several decades before the real effect of natural HRT in promoting or reducing different types of cancer will be known. The following reflects the current state of medical knowledge regarding the effect of HRT on the incidence of different types of cancer.

Endometrial and Ovarian Cancer

Modern combination HRT appears to reduce the risk of endometrial cancer, as well as that of ovarian cancer, perhaps by as much as 40 percent. This applies only if progesterone is taken for at least ten to fourteen days out of every monthly cycle. If only estrogen is taken, there is an increased risk of cancer of the uterus. This is why a woman who has a uterus must take progesterone in addition to estrogen. A woman taking combination HRT actually has less risk of developing uterine cancer than a woman who is not on HRT does.

Breast Cancer

Many women are reluctant to take HRT because they fear that it will increase their chances of developing breast cancer. This remains a complicated and controversial issue, especially as we are talking about the most common cancer in Western women. Statistics show that breast cancer affects one in every thirteen women by the age of seventy-five and one in eight women who have a family history of this disease (a mother or sister who has had breast cancer). In some cancerous tumors, a substance called estrogen-receptor protein is present, which increases the possibility that the cancer may be promoted by estrogen therapy.

The incidence of breast cancer continues to rise progressively throughout life, so one certainly would not want to do anything during midlife that might further increase this risk. Women who are most at risk of developing breast cancer include those who have never given birth or who were over thirty when they had their first children, obese women, women who went through puberty early (before the age of eleven) and/or who went through menopause late (after the age of fifty-four), and those with a family history of breast cancer. A common feature among these factors is a prolonged and constant exposure to estrogen from the ovaries. Women who eat diets high in fat and low in fiber have higher blood levels of estrogen than women on low-fat, high-fiber diets, and they also have a much higher incidence of breast cancer, so it seems that we have yet another possible link between estrogen and breast cancer.

Notwithstanding these theoretical considerations, however, of nearly thirty studies examining the relationship between estrogen replacement and breast cancer, the majority have failed to indicate a definitive for or against.[2] Individually, these studies have found either a small decrease or a small increase in the incidence of breast cancer in users of HRT. A widely publicized 1989 Swedish study linked estrogen with a slightly increased risk of breast cancer after six or more years of use. However, the conclusions were premature, as the researchers followed up on participants for an average duration of only 5.7 years, yet it is known that most breast cancers take seven years to grow large enough to be detected. Further, the same study found that when women using estrogen developed breast cancer, their survival rate was significantly better than that of women not on estrogen.

A very useful overview of twenty-three studies suggests that HRT neither increases nor decreases the incidence of breast cancer.[3] However, the results of studies on long-term (more than ten years) use of HRT counteract this finding and suggest that there may be a small increase in the risk of breast cancer. This increase is in the order of 1.3, which means that if you take estrogen replacement therapy for more than ten years, you may have a 30 percent increased risk of breast cancer.[4] Although the studies that show this increased risk are only population studies that surveyed women on HRT, rather than rigorously designed scientific trials comparing the experience of a group of women taking HRT with that of a group taking a placebo, they still should make a doctor cautious about prescribing high or prolonged doses of estrogen replacement therapy to a woman with a known high risk of breast cancer. In such a case, if estrogen therapy is necessary, I believe it is wise to use smaller or intermittent doses of estrogen replacement therapy. Long-term studies have also found that the risk of breast cancer does not increase until after at least five years of estrogen replacement therapy. This is reassuring for women who want to take estrogen replacement therapy for only a short time.[5]

In summary, with HRT of less than five years' duration, there is no increase in the incidence of breast cancer. The incidence may increase after ten to fifteen years of HRT, and this increase appears to be in the range of 30 percent. Furthermore, while it appears that the incidence of breast cancer may increase with long-term HRT, women who get breast cancer while on HRT are less likely to die from the disease.

As far as progesterone is concerned, there are some data to suggest that it offers some degree of protection against breast cancer in women on estrogen therapy, but the data as yet are inconclusive.

Skin Cancer

Studies suggest that the use of estrogen has no adverse effect on the subsequent development of malignant melanoma or other skin cancers. These cancers are primarily related to exposure to the sun's ultraviolet rays, rather than to hormonal factors.

In summary, it does not appear that properly balanced, natural HRT substantially increases the incidence of cancer. Moreover, the slight increase in the death rate from cancer is small compared to the reduction in the death rate from osteoporosis, heart disease, and stroke in estrogen users. Of course, statistics are a generalization, and an individual woman may not wish to base her personal decision about HRT on the results of studies of large population groups. In the final analysis, it is important that you feel good about your own decision regarding HRT. You need to trust your own instincts and judgment and those of your own doctor.

WHAT SHOULD I DO IF I HAVE IRREGULAR BLEEDING?

If you are taking HRT, it is normal for vaginal bleeding to occur within a few days of stopping the progestogen tablets. If bleeding starts while you are still taking the progestogen tablets, consult your doctor. It may need be necessary to change the dose or type of progestogen tablets. If bleeding occurs at any other time of the cycle, particularly when you are not taking your progestogen tablets, it can be a sign of a health problem such as a uterine polyp, uterine infection, fibroids, or uterine cancer. If you experience this type of abnormal irregular bleeding, you should see your gynecologist, who will undertake investigations to find the cause of bleeding. If tests show that all is well, you may continue taking HRT.

If you are postmenopausal (that is, if you have not had regular menstrual periods for twelve months) and you are *not* taking replacement hormones, you should consult your gynecologist about any bleeding from the vagina. The gynecologist will need to take samples of cells from the entire surface of the endometrium (the inner lining of the uterus) for testing, so that no areas are missed. To do this, your gynecologist may do a curettage or a hysteroscopy with directed endometrial biopsies. (For information about these procedures, see Chapter 3). With the hysteroscope, abnormal areas of the uterus can easily be seen, then biopsied (sampled) with a curette and sent to a laboratory for testing. Once this has been done, you will know whether or not your irregular bleeding is a sign of disease, and necessary treatment, if any, can be begun.

WILL I BECOME LESS FEMININE AFTER MENOPAUSE?

The menopausal ovary produces very little estrogen, but continues to make androgens, the so-called male sex hormones, which promote the development of masculine characteristics. This may cause a hormonal imbalance in which a menopausal woman has a relative excess of masculinizing hormones. In some women, this may result in an increase in the amount of facial hair, thinning of the scalp hair, coarsening of the skin and facial features, shrinkage of the breasts, and a slight deepening of the voice. This is not inevitable, however, and there are measures you can take to combat these unpleasant symptoms. (See What Can I Do If I Have Too Many Male Hormones? on page 88 for a summary of available strategies.)

In most cases, such hormonal imbalances can easily be fixed by simply taking natural estrogen replacement. This increases the amount of feminizing hormones in your body and at the same time reduces the production of masculinizing hormones in the ovaries. This will greatly lessen the development of masculine features.

If estrogen replacement alone is not sufficient to prevent excessive growth of facial hair or thinning of the scalp hair, it may be necessary to use a special hormone commonly called an "anti-male hormone." Spironolactone (also sold under the brand name Aldactone) is one variety of anti-male hormone. Many women find that spironolactone, taken either by itself or in combination with natural estrogen, is sufficient to control excessive facial and body hair as well as acne. Spironolactone takes six to twelve months to be really effective in controlling these symptoms of excessive masculinizing hormones.

Another anti-male hormone is cyproterone acetate (sold under the brand name Androcur), which reduces the production and action of masculinizing hormones in the body. It also acts like progesterone and can be prescribed along with estrogen to regulate and balance menstrual blood flow. Cyproterone acetate is extremely effective, but, unfortunately, it has not yet been approved by the U.S. Food and Drug Administration, so it is not readily available in the United States. It is, however, available in Canada, as well as in Europe, Australia, and South Africa, where it is commonly prescribed by doctors for women with excessive amounts of masculinizing hormones. Your doctor may be able to obtain it for you if he or she applies to the FDA for permission to use it for research purposes. It is also known that quite a large amount of Androcur crosses the Canadian/American border for use by American women, so you might discuss this alternative with your doctor.

If you find unwelcome masculine changes occurring in your body but do not want to take hormonal therapy, there is no need for you to feel that you cannot look and feel feminine. Facial and body hair can be controlled with electrolysis, bleaching, waxing, and/or shaving. A body wave or permanent can make thinning scalp hair seem fuller. A good skin care routine and the use of products such as facial peels and masks can refine and improve the complexion. Consult a good beautician, hairdresser, or skin care specialist. In Chapter 6, I will discuss certain foods that are natural sources of plant estrogens. Try to eat more of these foods regularly, as these are both slimming and feminizing. By paying attention to nutrition and exercise, keeping your weight in the healthy range, and wearing attractive clothing and jewelry, you can feel and look very much like an attractive woman. Keep in mind, too, that your mental attitude is very important. A woman who is physically and mentally active and enthusiastic will be seen as feminine and attractive by herself and by others.

WHAT IF MY MENOPAUSE IS EARLY?

Premature menopause is defined as menopause that occurs before the age of forty years. Often, the cause of premature menopause—also called early ovarian failure—cannot be determined. However, factors that may play a role are heredity, stress, heavy smoking, poor diet, excessive alcohol consumption, and autoimmune diseases (diseases caused by imbalances or malfunctions in the immune system). A woman who undergoes menopause prematurely may have been born with fewer eggs in her ovaries; if they are released at the normal rate, her eggs would soon be depleted. Radiation therapy for pelvic cancer, or chemotherapy for any type of cancer, can quickly destroy a large number of eggs, leaving an insufficient number to last for very long. A severe infection of the ovaries caused by a viral illness such as mumps can also damage large numbers of eggs. In some cases, the ovaries simply become dormant, and although there may be enough eggs, they refuse to respond normally to follicle-stimulating hormone and so they fail to produce estrogen. This may be temporary and the ovaries may come back into action, or it may be permanent. Surgical removal of the ovaries before the age of forty will bring on a sudden and severe premature menopause if hormone replacement is not taken.

Women who experience premature menopause, no matter what the cause, are at early and increased risk for developing cardiovascular disease and osteoporosis. To prevent these debilitating diseases, unless she has another health problem that would prohibit it, a woman who has a premature menopause should take sufficient HRT at the time of her menopause, and ideally up to the age of fifty—in some cases, even longer, especially if her bone density is low. This should give her adequate protection.

A woman who goes through premature menopause frequently experiences a wide range of negative emotions, including anger, disbelief, shock, resentment, and shame. If you are in this situation,

What Can I Do If I Have Too Many "Male" Hormones?

Excessive activity of masculinizing hormones (especially the free male hormones testosterone, androstenedione, and dehydroepiandrosterone) in your body may produce unsightly facial or body hair, baldness, and acne. Fortunately, we have ways to control these annoying problems.

I have developed five different hormonal regimens for relieving these symptoms. Your doctor can adapt any of these to suit your particular needs:

1. *For mild cases, natural estrogen alone may be sufficient (if you have your uterus, you will also need to take progesterone).*

2. *If estrogen alone is insufficient, a regimen of natural estrogen plus 50 to 200 milligrams of spironolactone (Aldactone) daily may be effective.*

3. *If you are unable to tolerate estrogen, spironolactone can be taken by itself.*

4. *A cortisone-type drug, taken in a small dosage (0.25 milligrams of dexamethasone, for example) at night may be helpful.*

5. *Another alternative is a regimen of natural estrogen daily, plus 2.5 to 100 milligrams of cyproterone acetate (Androcur) daily for three weeks of every month. This requires that you have access to a doctor who is working with Androcur under an investigational exemption from the FDA, or that you obtain a referral to a doctor in a country where it is approved for general use. (See page 86).*

There are also a number of nonhormonal strategies that can be helpful. Consult the table on the next page to learn about your options.

Problem	Strategies
Excessive facial and body hair	Under the supervision of a beautician, try one or more of the following:
	• Waxing (but not for very coarse, thick hair).
	• Bleaching (for mustache).
	• Depilatory creams.
	• Shaving (contrary to popular belief, shaving does not increase hair regrowth).
	• Electrolysis (for small areas only)
	Plucking is not recommended.
Balding; hair loss on scalp	Ask your doctor to check the function of your thyroid gland (an underactive thyroid can cause hair loss). Nutritional supplements can help greatly. Take 1,000 mg of calcium, 500 mg of magnesium, and 30 mg of zinc chelate daily, as well as trace minerals such as manganese, boron, silica, iodine, iron, chromium, and molybdenum. Take 3000 mg of evening primrose oil daily. Consider having a permanent or body wave to make hair appear fuller.
Acne	Use an herbal skin peel or clay-based mask product several times weekly or as needed. Keep your skin scrupulously clean. Use only noncomedogenic (non-pore-clogging) cosmetics and skin care products. Take 500 IU of vitamin A, 500 IU of vitamin E, 2,000 mg of vitamin C, and 30 mg of zinc chelate daily. Ask your doctor about a prescription for topical tretinoin (Retin-A cream), which also has anti-aging effects.

it is important that you receive counseling from a sympathetic doctor or qualified therapist, because if you bottle up these feelings, you may find yourself feeling very depressed.

If you have a very early menopause—say, when you are under the age of thirty—you may find it difficult to relate to much of the information available about menopause, which is usually designed with fifty-year-old women in mind, and thus you may find yourself feeling increasingly isolated. However, if you can find an understanding doctor, you should be able to work through these negative feelings. It is important to understand that menopause is *not* synonymous with old age. If you go through menopause early, it merely means that your ovaries have exhausted their supply of eggs sooner than normal.

A premature menopause, if properly treated, will not cause you to age more quickly, or to change your personality or mental ability. Indeed, to all your friends and family, you will appear just the same as before. When it comes to your sex life, adequate HRT should help you to feel and act just as sexy as ever. (For information about sex and menopause, see Chapter 8.) You may, however, need larger doses or a different form of HRT than a woman of fifty or sixty.

IF I HAVE A PREMATURE MENOPAUSE, CAN I HAVE CHILDREN?

Generally, by the time premature menopause is diagnosed, a woman's fertility is very low. It is often too late to successfully restimulate ovulation, even with the use of fertility drugs. However, that doesn't necessarily mean you have to give up hope of becoming a mother. Adoption is one possibility. Recently, the option of obtaining a donor egg or embryo has also become possible. Donor eggs and embryos enable women who do not have a living supply of their own eggs to have the chance of a lifetime.

Normally, an egg donor is a close relative, and both the donor and the prospective mother must take part in an in vitro fertilization (IVF) program. The donor's ovaries are hyperstimulated to produce a crop of premium eggs. The eggs are collected and then fertilized in vitro (in a test tube), usually with the recipient's partner's sperm. The resulting embryo is then implanted into the menopausal woman's uterus, which has been suitably prepared with hormone therapy. If no relative is available to serve as a donor, spare donor eggs or embryos from an unrelated person who is going through the IVF program may be available. Egg and embryo donation has been fairly successful, with up to a 20- to 40-percent chance of a normal pregnancy for women who become pregnant this way.

Yes, it is amazing to think that egg donation offers menopausal women of any age the possibility to become pregnant and have a baby. I wonder if in the future we will see more women in their fifties and sixties having maternal urges?

AT THE END OF THE DAY, IS HRT REALLY SAFE?

Thus far, our experience using hormone replacement therapy in large

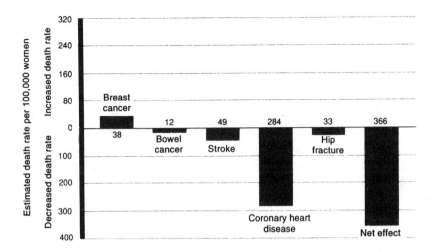

Figure 5.1 Hormone Replacement Therapy and Its Relative Risks

This diagram shows the anticipated effect of HRT on the number of deaths from heart disease, osteoporosis, and certain types of cancer, based on the difference in the number of deaths from these diseases in a sample of 100,000 women who took HRT for a period of ten years and that in a comparable group of women who did not take HRT.

numbers of women has produced some interesting statistics. If we look at all the major studies done so far and try to be as honest as we can (if not a little pessimistic), the overall results come out in favor of HRT, as its benefits outweigh its risks. Statistically, if we took 100,000 women and gave them estrogen replacement therapy for ten years, we would expect that 38 more of them would get breast cancer than would have otherwise; however, 366 women would be saved from stroke, heart disease, and osteoporotic fractures.[6] In other words, more lives would be saved than lost by long-term HRT. Figure 5.1 shows this diagrammatically.

But the idea of treating all menopausal women with HRT remains controversial, especially as this would mean treating women with no symptoms and no risk factors for osteoporosis or cardiovascular disease. It is easy to understand why many menopausal women feel confused, when controversy and disagreement exist among the medical profession. Some women feel that they don't want to be part of a generation of "hormone guinea pigs." Of course, 100 years from now, we will have more conclusive evidence if taking HRT saves lives—but you may not want to wait that long!

Nothing in life can promise to be perfect. The best that today's woman can do is to seek the best compromise or balance among all her options. At the end of the day, it is you who must decide what is best for your individual lifestyle and long-term health.

Whether you decide to take HRT or not, you should see your doctor at least annually for the rest of your life, as your medical needs often change over the years. Furthermore, your risk of cancer, cardiovascular disease, and osteoporosis rises with increasing age. By visiting your doctor regularly, these degenerative diseases can be detected early and thus treated more effectively. In many cases, their progression can be prevented by regular supervision and treatment or modification of diet and lifestyle.

Chapter 6

NATUROPATHIC MEDICINE FOR MENOPAUSE

For twenty years I have prescribed various combinations of vitamins, minerals, essential fatty acids, and herbs, in addition to orthodox medicines, to help women achieve optimum well-being during the menopausal years. The tremendous difference these nutritional supplements can make never ceases to impress me, and I firmly believe that using them is worth any extra effort and expense.

Many women prefer the process of menopause to be a natural one. The good news is that there are naturopathic means of easing many menopausal discomforts, including hot flashes, dryness and wrinkling of the skin, anxiety, and stress, as well as of improving the overall functioning of the immune system. There are also effective natural strategies for preventing or slowing the progression of some of the longer term consequences of estrogen deficiency, such as cardiovascular disease and osteoporosis. Even if you take hormone replacement therapy, dietary modification, nutritional and dietary supplements, herbs, and other naturopathic approaches can be used to great advantage.

NATURAL THERAPIES FOR THE SYMPTOMS OF MENOPAUSE

Many of the discomforts of the menopausal period can be helped with simple, natural treatments that you can use at home, such as increasing your consumption of foods that contain natural plant estrogens, drinking adequate amounts of water, taking selected nutritional supplements, and using specific herbs. Table 6.1 gives an overview of the nutritional and dietary supplements, herbs, and other measures recommended for some of the most common menopausal symptoms.

You can choose to use one, several, or all of the therapies recommended, and you can use these natural treatments either alone or in combination with hormone replacement therapy.

Natural Plant Estrogens

Over 300 different plants contain estrogenic substances. Although these are weak estrogens and are present only in tiny quantities, if foods containing them are consumed regularly, they can exert a mild estrogenic effect in humans.[1]

Alfalfa contains a plant estrogen called coumestrol, which can actually cause infertility in animals that graze on large pastures of alfalfa grasses. Of all the plant estrogens, coumestrol is the most potent, although it is still 200 times weaker than human estrogens. The herb red clover also contains coumestrol and can be taken in the form of an herbal tea, or you can make fresh sprouts from red clover seeds. As some varieties of red clover are poisonous, however, it is best to obtain supplies from a reputable herbalist or health food store. Soybeans, soybean sprouts, and flaxseed meal (crushed flaxseeds) are excellent sources of natural estrogens as well as of protein and essential fatty acids. They are definitely anti-aging foods for menopausal women. For a list of foods and herbs that are good sources of plant estrogens, see Foods Containing Natural Estrogens on page 98.

Natural plant estrogens provide a useful form of estrogen supplementation for women who are unable to or who choose not to take estrogen replacement therapy. Because these plant estrogens are low in potency, they are safe and will not produce the side effects sometimes seen with HRT. If you want to boost your estrogen level, I suggest you eat approximately two cups daily of foods listed on page 98—for example, two cups of mixed sprouts, parsley, soybeans, legumes, and fennel, along with a wide selection of fresh vegetables. Make sure you vary your sources of plant estrogens by using different foods each day to make up your two cups' worth of estrogenic foods.

Plant estrogens are also present in bourbon, whiskey, gin, ouzo, and beer. These estrogens are partly responsible for the breast development seen in alcoholic males, as their damaged livers are unable to break down and inactivate the estrogens found in alcoholic beverages. However, I do not recommend that you try to increase your estrogen level by drinking alcohol.

Table 6.1 Naturopathic Strategies for Symptoms of Menopause

The following table offers suggestions for herbs, dietary supplements, and other natural strategies that are helpful for common menopausal symptoms. Note that the dosages for some of the items recommended are given in milligrams (mg), some in micrograms (mcg), and some in international units (IU). Both milligrams and micrograms are measures of weight (1 milligram is equal to 1,000 micrograms). International units are measures of the activity of a substance, not its weight; the number of milligrams or micrograms in an international unit therefore varies, depending on the substance being measured. Note also that appropriate doses of herbs may vary depending on the individual; if you have any doubts, consult a qualified herbalist or naturopathic physician for a personalized herbal prescription.

Problem	Strategies
Hot flashes, sweating	Drink 2 quarts (8 glasses) of water daily. Take 1,000 mg of evening primrose oil and 100 IU of vitamin E, three times a day. Take one or more of the following herbs daily: • 1,000 mg of dong quai. • 500–1,000 mg of licorice (or 1–2 cups of licorice tea). • 500–1,000 mg of black cohosh. • 500–1,000 mg of sarsaparilla (or 2–3 cups of sarsaparilla tea). • 300–600 mg of chaste tree (*Vitex agnus-castus*). *Note:* Licorice can elevate blood pressure. If you have high blood presure, use it with caution or avoid it entirely.
Dry, itchy skin; vaginal dryness	Drink 2 quarts (8 glasses) of water daily. Take 1,000 mg of evening primrose oil, three times a day. Take the following antioxidant supplements (with food): • 5,000 IU of vitamin A *or* 10 mg of beta-carotene, once daily. • 500 IU of vitamin E, once daily. • 50 mcg of selenium, once daily. • 1,000–2,000 mg of vitamin C with bioflavonoids, three times daily. Use only cold-pressed vegetable oils such as olive, flaxseed, grape seed, canola, and sesame oils in cooking and salad dressings.

Problem	Strategies
Fatigue, poor memory, reduced mental efficiency	Take a balanced high-potency vitamin B complex tablet or capsule daily. Take 1,000 mg of evening primrose oil, three times a day. Take 1,000 mg of ginkgo biloba, 1,000–4,000 mg of ginseng, and/or 1,000 mg of royal jelly daily.
Anxiety, irritability, mood disorders, insomnia	Take one or more of the following herbs daily (take them at bedtime for insomnia): • 250 mg of passion flower. • 1,000 mg of valerian root (or 2 cups of valerian root tea). • 1–2 cups of lime flower tea. • 1–2 tablespoons of oats. • 500 mg of skullcap. Take 4,000 mg of lecithin and 500–1,500 mg of the amino acid L-glutamine daily. Take a balanced high-potency vitamin B complex tablet or capsule daily, plus additional amounts of the following: • 500 mg of vitamin B_5 (pantothenic acid). • 500 mg of choline. • 50 mg of vitamin B_6 (pyridoxine). Take 500 mg of magnesium (as magnesium chelate) daily.
Muscle and joint aches and pains, degenerative diseases of the bones, muscles, and joints	Take 1,000 mg of evening primrose oil, three times daily. Take 1,000 mg of fish oil daily. Take the following antioxidant supplements daily: • 10,000 IU of vitamin A *or* 20 mg of beta-carotene. • 2,000 mg of vitamin C (in mineral ascorbate form with bioflavonoids). • 500 IU of vitamin E. Take the following minerals: • 1,000 mg of calcium at bedtime. • 500 mg of magnesium at bedtime. • 1.5–3.0 mg of copper daily. • 20 mg of boron (as sodium borate) daily. • 25 mg of silica daily. • 10 mg of manganese (as manganese chelate) daily. • 30 mg of zinc (as zinc chelate) daily. Take 400 IU of vitamin D_3 (cholecalciferol) and 100 mcg of vitamin K daily.

Problem	Strategies
Rapid aging of the skin, thinning hair, brittle nails, osteoporosis	Take 1,000 mg of calcium and 500 mg of magnesium at bedtime. Take the following vitamins daily: • 5,000 IU of vitamin A *or* 20 mg of beta-carotene. • 2,000 mg of vitamin C, preferably in mineral ascorbate form with bioflavonoids. • 500 IU of vitamin E. • 400 IU of vitamin D_3 (cholecalciferol). • 100 mcg of vitamin K. Take the following trace minerals daily: • 20 mg of boron (as sodium borate). • 5 mg of copper (as copper chelate). • 30 mg of zinc (as zinc chelate). • 25 mg of silica. • 10 mg of manganese (as manganese chelate).

Water

Many women find the drinking of pure water a chore and do it grudgingly, much like a penance. It is an acquired habit, but once you start drinking between one and two quarts of pure water daily, your body will soon crave it if you forget. Just think how tired and sad plants look without water. Well, we are just the same!

You may flavor your water with herbal teas or a dash of fresh citrus fruit, but otherwise leave it pure, so that it can act as a cleanser and detoxifier. There is no other cleanser like water. I see many women in their middle years with conditions such as joint pains, bad breath, and osteoarthritis, who did not start drinking adequate amounts of water until it was too late.

Start today. Drink at least one and a half quarts of pure water, gradually, throughout the morning and afternoon. Keep a jug of water on your desk or carry a water bottle with you on your travels. It's well worth the extra trips to the bathroom! By drinking cool water regularly you will reduce hot flashes, headaches, joint pains, fatigue, and dry, itchy skin, and you will rejuvenate your entire cardiovascular system.

Nutritional and Dietary Supplements

There are a number of nutritional and dietary supplements that are especially useful to women who are going through menopause. In addition to supporting overall health, certain nutrients can actually

Foods Containing Natural Estrogens

A number of different foods and herbs are sources of natural plant estrogens, and can be very helpful during menopause. The following is a list of some of the best food sources of estrogen. These foods not only contain estrogens, but are high in vitamins, minerals, fiber, and essential fatty acids, and they are low in saturated fat. Thus, there are many good reasons to consume them on a regular basis.

- Alfalfa
- Anise seed
- Apples
- Baker's yeast
- Barley
- Beets
- Cabbage
- Carrots
- Cherries
- Chickpeas
- Clover
- Corn
- Corn oil
- Cowpeas (black-
  eyed peas)
- Cucumbers

- Fennel
- Flaxseeds
- Garlic
- Green beans
- Green squash
- Hops
- Licorice
- Oats
- Olive oil
- Olives
- Papaya
- Parsley
- Peas
- Plums
- Potatoes
- Pumpkin

- Red beans
- Red clover
- Rhubarb
- Rice
- Rye
- Sage
- Sesame seeds
- Soybean sprouts
- Soybeans
- Split peas
- Squash
- Sunflower seeds
- Wheat
- Yams

help to relieve unpleasant symptoms. The supplements I recommend include vitamins, minerals, amino acids, and essential fatty acids.

Vitamin A

Vitamin A has many essential roles in the body. It is required for night vision, a healthy immune system, and reproduction. It is also an antioxidant. (For information about vitamin A's role as an antioxidant, see Chapter 7).

Persons lacking in vitamin A may develop skin and mucous membrane disorders in which the tissues become white, hard, and chronically inflamed. This makes them more susceptible to infection.

Vitamin A comes in two forms: preformed vitamin A (retinol or retinyl esters), which is found in cod and halibut liver, cream, butter, eggs, and animal meats and livers; and provitamin A (beta-carotene), which is found in sweet potatoes, papayas, apricots, watermelons, and tomatoes, and in green, yellow, and orange vegetables. The liver converts beta-carotene into vitamin A as the body needs it.

Both vitamin A and beta-carotene strengthen mucous membranes throughout the body. This is helpful for the unpleasant menopausal symptoms of vaginal dryness and fragility. I have found that the combination of vitamin A (or beta-carotene) and evening primrose oil is effective in reducing the itchy, crawling sensation in the skin that often occurs during menopause.

The U.S. recommended daily allowance of vitamin A is 5,000 international units. However, smokers, regular drinkers of alcohol, junk-food consumers, diabetics, and those exposed to excessive pollutants and toxic chemicals often need more. If you have dry and irritated skin and mucous membranes, it is safe to take 10,000 international units of vitamin A or 20,000 to 25,000 international units of beta-carotene daily. Doses above 10,000 international units of vitamin A daily should not be taken without medical supervision, as very high doses (25,000 to 50,000 international units daily) can be toxic. A pregnant woman should never take more than 5,000 international units of vitamin A daily.

Unlike vitamin A, beta-carotene is nontoxic, even in high doses, so there is no need to worry about overdosage. However, no more than 25,000 international units daily is needed to achieve maximal benefits.

The B Vitamins

The B vitamins are a vital group of nutrients that are involved in the functioning of the nervous system and in maintaining healthy skin, eyes, and hair. They also support adrenal gland function and are involved in energy production. The B vitamins should always be taken as a group, in a balanced B complex supplement. If you take any of the B vitamins individually, you should also take a B complex supplement at a different time of day.

Vitamin B5 (pantothenic acid), vitamin B6 (pyridoxine), and choline are three simple and inexpensive nutrients that can neatly provide help for the common menopausal symptoms of anxiety, poor sleep, and loss of libido. Vitamin B6 is required for the conversion of amino acids into neurotransmitters (brain chemicals). In particular, B6 is essential for the conversion of the amino acid tryptophan into the neurotransmitter serotonin. Serotonin exerts an antidepressant effect, and normal amounts are required for a healthy libido. The recommended daily dose of vitamin B6 is 50 to 100 milligrams. Do not take more than this, or transient nerve damage can occur. Good food sources of vitamin B6 are meats, whole grains, and brewer's yeast.

Vitamin B5 and choline are the precursors for the neurotransmitter acetylcholine. Acetylcholine is required for the normal functioning of memory. People who suffer from anxiety often have excessive levels of adrenline and insufficient amounts of acetylcholine in their bodies. Acetylcholine is one of the neurotransmitters required for the action of the autonomic nervous system, which is involved in sexual excitement and orgasm. Ensuring adequate levels of acetylcholine helps to maintain sexual responsiveness and enjoyment of lovemaking. The recommended dose of both vitamin B5 and choline is 500 milligrams daily. Vitamin B5 is present organ meats, eggs, and whole grain cereals. Good food sources of choline include lecithin, eggs, soybeans, cauliflower, cabbage, tofu, and tempeh.

Vitamin C

Vitamin C, or ascorbic acid, is so vital to human health that I have often thought it to be an evolutionary defect that the human body does not manufacture its own supply. Most animals produce their own supplies of vitamin C, which increase when they are under stress.

Vitamin C was made famous by the research of the late Dr. Linus Pauling. Dr. Pauling, twice a Nobel laureate, stated that vitamin C could prevent the common cold and treat cancer. Many doctors believe that vitamin C can reduce the severity of colds and help prevent cancer, although it cannot control established, advanced cancers. Still other doctors do not believe in using nutritional supplements at all—generally because university medical schools are only just starting to include in their curricula any study of nutrition as a therapeutic tool.

Vitamin C is needed for the manufacture of collagen, which acts like a flexible or elastic protein glue in connective tissue and bone. Ensuring plentiful vitamin C helps to maintain healthy collagen, thereby keeping the skin and mucous membranes thicker and stronger and the skeleton more flexible. If your ligaments and bones are more flexible, they are less likely to be torn (sprained) or broken (fractured). Vitamin C is also a powerful antioxidant and free-radical scavenger that helps to reduce degenerative diseases and inflammation, and to slow down the aging process. (For information about the role of vitamin C as an antioxidant, see Chapter 7).

Vitamin C is found in high concentrations in the brain and the adrenal glands, and it is required for these organs to function under stress. I always recommend that people who are under mental or physical stress take additional vitamin C, and have found it to have a natural relaxing effect.

The recommended dose of vitamin C is quite a controversial subject among doctors. Although many agree that the U.S. recommended daily allowance of 60 milligrams is inadequate for optimal health, few agree with Dr. Pauling that the daily requirement is between 2,000 and 9,000 milligrams. What is true is that the daily requirement for vitamin C varies greatly among individuals. Factors that increase a person's daily requirement are stress, smoking, infections, surgery, exposure to pollution, and the consumption of alcohol. If you do not eat fresh *raw* fruits and vegetables every day, you may be deficient in vitamin C, as the body is continually using it up. Vitamin C is destroyed by high temperatures, which is why raw foods are so important.

I believe it is imperative to get at least 1,000 milligrams daily, and if any factors that increase your need, such as those mentioned above, are present, you may require up to 6,000 milligrams daily. It is best to take it in divided doses, *with* food. However, it is much better to get your vitamin C from natural, fresh raw food sources than to rely on supplements alone. Good food sources of vitamin C include citrus fruits, tomatoes, capsicum, Brussels sprouts, broccoli, berries (blueberries, gooseberries, raspberries, strawberries), bananas, alfalfa, guava, kidney, oysters, potatoes, cantaloupe, sweet potatoes, spinach, watermelon, green leafy vegetables, green and red peppers, sprouted grains, and rose hips.

In most of the high-vitamin-C foods, there are also other nutrients, called bioflavonoids (or, occasionally, vitamin P). There are around 500 different bioflavonoids found in food plants. Bioflavonoids aid in the absorption and utilization of vitamin C and enhance its antioxidant properties. Some vitamin C supplements contain bioflavonoids as well.

Vitamin D

Vitamin D, or cholecalciferol, functions as both a vitamin and a hormone. Vitamin D is synthesized in the skin when the skin is exposed to the sun's ultraviolet rays. It is required for the absorption and utilization of calcium and helps calcium to be deposited in your bones. Gross deficiencies of vitamin D cause osteomalacia, which is a bone demineralizing disease not unlike osteoporosis. Osteomalacia is the adult equivalent of childhood rickets. Even marginal or slight deficiencies of vitamin D can increase your risk of osteoporosis and deterioration of the joints. Deficiencies of vitamin D can also contribute to thinning of the hair, brittleness of the nails, and rapid aging of the skin.

Vitamin D is not present in a wide variety of foods, but is confined mainly to fish liver oils, fatty fish, liver, egg yolks, and butter, and, to a lesser degree, cow's milk. It is not unusual for women to be deficient in vitamin D, as many of us now avoid the sun and at the same time, in our constant effort to lose weight, we are reducing the amount of eggs, dairy products, and fatty fish we eat. Those who have difficulty digesting and absorbing fats can easily develop suboptimal levels of vitamin D. Your doctor can test you for vitamin D deficiency with a simple blood test.

The U.S. recommended daily allowance of vitamin D is 400 international units. Supplements of 200 to 400 international units daily are a good idea if you avoid sunlight and fatty foods. Take vitamin D supplements with meals or drink vitamin-D-fortified milk. Do not take excessive doses of vitamin D, however, as this may cause very high blood calcium levels, calcifications in the body's soft tissues and organs, and kidney stones. Doses less than 1,000 international units daily are considered most unlikely to exert any dangerous effects. Even so, if you have a tendency to develop kidney stones, you should take vitamin D or calcium supplements only under medical supervision.

Vitamin E

Vitamin E is essential for the existence of all oxygen-breathing creatures. It has a protective, or sparing, effect on estrogen, so that your estrogen (whether your own or from hormone replacement therapy) lasts longer. As a result, vitamin E helps to reduce hot flashes. Some women have told me that vitamin E supplements delayed menopause and the state of estrogen deficiency. Perhaps the ancient Greeks knew of the hormonal benefits of eating foods high in vitamin E; the chemical name for vitamin E is *tocopherol*, which in Greek means "to carry and bear babies."

Together with vitamin A, vitamin E strengthens the skin and mucous membranes. Many women find that these vitamins reduce vaginal dryness and shrinkage. Vitamin E also reduces free radical damage to your cells' membranes and is a poweful anti-aging nutrient. (For information about the actions of vitamin E as an antioxidant, see Chapter 7).

The recommended daily dose of vitamin E is from 100 to 500 international units daily. Start slowly, gradually building up the dosage, to avoid a sudden boost to your cardiovascular system. Over the long term, daily doses of 100 international units are generally sufficient. If you find brown age spots appearing on your skin, taking additional vitamin E can reverse this degenerative process. Take 500 international units daily until the spots fade, and apply a combination of vitamin E cream and aloe vera gel to the affected areas twice daily.

Vitamin K

Vitamin K is a fat-soluble vitamin that is needed for the synthesis of several blood-clotting factors, and for this reason it can reduce the heavy menstrual bleeding that is common in the perimenopausal years. Vitamin K is also needed for the mineralization of bone and helps to keep your bones stronger and more resilient to breakage. Some preliminary studies suggest that vitamin K can be significant in the prevention of osteoporosis.

Vitamin K deficiency is not common, as this nutrient is present in many different types of foods, and bacteria in the intestines synthesize a large proportion of daily vitamin K requirements. If you take antibiotics frequently, however, you can greatly reduce your production of vitamin K. A tendency to bruise easily can be a sign of vitamin K deficiency.

The recommended daily allowance for vitamin K is 65 micrograms, an amount that normally is easily obtained in the diet. Good food sources include green leafy vegetables, egg yolks, blackstrap molasses, alfalfa, kelp, nettles, dairy products, wheat bran, wheat germ, soybean oil, and cod liver oil. Foods containing lactobacillus bacteria (such as kefir, whey, and yogurt) add friendly bacteria that produce vitamin K to the intestines. If you have malabsorption or digestive problems, or take antibiotics frequently, a supplement of 50 to 100 micrograms daily is desirable.

Boron

Boron is a trace mineral found in plant foods, and its health benefits are becoming increasingly evident. A study done in 1987 found that boron may be helpful in preventing osteoporosis.[2] Twelve post-menopausal women between the ages of forty-eight and eighty-two were studied for twenty-four weeks. During the first seventeen weeks, they were given a diet low in boron (which is what many women normally consume), and during the subsequent seven weeks they received 3 milligrams of boron daily.

Eight days after they began taking boron, the women's urinary losses of calcium and magnesium were greatly reduced, and they had significant increases (approximately twofold) in their production of estrogen and testosterone. Reducing the loss of magnesium from the body is very desirable, as magnesium is essential for a healthy cardiovascular system and skeleton. This research suggests that taking boron supplements, especially if your dietary intake of boron is low, can cause favorable changes in mineral metabolism that can reduce, and may even prevent, the loss of mineral from the bones (osteoporosis). Boron is also necessary for healthy hair, skin, and nails, and an adequate intake of boron may help prevent muscle and joint aches and pains.

Foods high in boron include fruits, vegetables, and sesame seeds. Meats and poultry, on the other hand, are low in boron. Boron is available in supplement form, most commonly as sodium borate. An appropriate dosage would be 5 to 20 milligrams daily.

Calcium

As discussed in Chapter 2, many perimenopausal women do not consume the recommended daily allowance of 1,000 milligrams of calcium. This can increase their risk of developing osteoporosis, cardiovascular disease, arthritis, cramps, and fragile skin. Calcium and magnesium work together to form bone substance and to regulate muscular tone, and they are required in a ratio of 2 to 1 (that is, 200 milligrams of calcium per 100 milligrams of magnesium). Every woman should consume at least 1,000 milligrams of calcium per day, either from food sources or in supplement form (see page 121).

Copper

Copper is an essential trace mineral. Together with iron, copper enables the blood protein hemoglobin to carry precious oxygen to your cells.

Copper is a component in superoxide dismutase, an antioxidant enzyme produced by the body that protects against damage from free radicals. Copper is bound to the protein ceruloplasmin, which is a very important antioxidant in the blood. Ceruloplasmin prevents peroxidation (rancidity) of the polyunsaturated fats in cell membranes. An adequate intake of copper is also needed for healthy skin, hair, nails, and bones. It is involved in the production of collagen, a tough, fibrous, yet elastic, tissue found in bone, tendons, skin, and cartilage. Indeed, copper is a known folk remedy for arthritis; some people swear by their copper bracelets.

Symptoms of copper deficiency include anemia, osteoporosis, and brittle, inflexible bones. There is a wide variation in dietary copper intake, and many women may be getting sub-optimal amounts. This may not cause obvious symptoms, but it is a concern, given copper's vital role in maintaining bone and ligament integrity and in forming antioxidant reserves.

Good food sources of copper are animal liver, crustaceans, nuts, oysters, legumes, kidneys, fruits, and shellfish. You can also take copper in supplement form, as copper gluconate, copper sulfate, or copper amino acid chelate. The recommended dose is 1.5 to 3 milligrams daily. The ratio of copper to zinc taken in supplement form should be 1 to 10; that is, if you take 30 milligrams of zinc, then the required dose of copper is 3 milligrams. However, if you have Wilson's disease—a rare hereditary syndrome characterized by an inability to metabolize copper properly—you should not take any copper supplements.

Magnesium

Magnesium is a mineral that has many important functions in the body. Among other things, it is involved in the production of enzymes and in the process by which cellular energy is released. Because it plays an important role in regulating muscular tone, it can serve as a natural muscle relaxant, making it useful for relieving such symptoms as muscle cramping and anxiety. Many menopausal women suffer from heart palpitations (an irregular or racing heartbeat) associated with hot flashes. This can be helped by increasing your intake of magnesium. Magnesium and calcium supplementation, in a ratio of 2 milligrams of calcium for each milligram of magnesium, can reduce bone loss after menopause. Magnesium is also essential for the health of the heart and the circulatory system (see page 121). An appropriate supplemental dose of magnesium is around 500 milligrams daily.

Manganese

Manganese is a vital mineral for health and is required for the metabolism of food and the production of sex hormones. Like copper, it is an antioxidant and is an element in superoxide dismutase, a potent antioxidant enzyme, and thus helps to reduce degenerative diseases associated with aging. Manganese is also part of normal bone and cartilage structure, and can be helpful for sufferers of osteoarthritis. Some studies have found that women with osteoporosis have low levels of manganese compared with women whose bones are normal.

The National Research Council of America states that an adequate daily intake of manganese is 2 to 5 milligrams, and that up to 10 milligrams daily is safe. Good food sources of manganese are whole grains and nuts, wheat bran, organ meats, shellfish, and milk. Many fruits and vegetables contain moderate amounts, but this varies depending on the manganese content of the soil where they were grown. Manganese can be taken in supplement form as manganese gluconate or manganese amino acid chelate.

Selenium

Selenium is a trace mineral that is vital for good health. It is important in maintaining healthy immune function and tissue elasticity, including that of the skin and mucous membranes. It is also an important antioxidant that works synergistically with vitamin E to prevent free radical damage and support the health of the heart and circulatory system. (For information about the antioxidant actions of selenium, see Chapter 7).

Silica

Silica is a form of the mineral silicon, which is the second most abundant element in the earth's outer layer. Silicon is used to make glass and computer chips, among other things, and in the last decade has been found to be an essential trace mineral for animals and for humans.

Silicon is found in human bone, fingernails, skin, and connective tissue, and adds mechanical integrity and hardness to their architectural matrix. Some researchers believe that silicon may offer some protection against atherosclerosis by strengthening connective tissue in the blood vessel walls.

The best food sources of silicon and silica are seafoods, whole grains, and vegetables. If you consume a balanced diet, you probably get about 200 milligrams of silica daily. The herb horsetail is high in silica, and can be taken as a tea or in the form of an extract called vegetal silica. Silica can also be taken as part of a multimineral formula. Taking moderate amounts of supplemental silica has no known side effects. The recommended dosage is 25 to 100 milligrams daily.

Zinc

Zinc is an essential mineral for the body, as more than 200 enzymes require zinc for their activity. It is also important for the proper functioning of cell membranes. Zinc is vital for a healthy immune system and helps to keep hair, nails, and bones strong.

Good food sources of zinc include brewer's yeast, seafoods, whole grain products, wheat bran, lean meats, blackstrap molasses, liver, sesame and sunflower seeds, and oatmeal. Zinc can also be taken in supplement form as zinc amino acid chelate. Recommended supplemental doses for women are 15 to 30 milligrams daily. To avoid possible stomach upset, take zinc supplements with food, and do not exceed the recommended dosage, as the consumption of too much zinc may upset the balance of other necessary minerals in the body. It is best to take zinc on an intermittent basis, for example, three months on, three months off.

L-Glutamine

L-glutamine is an amino acid that crosses the blood-brain barrier and passes into the brain tissue, where it is converted into glutamic acid. The brain then converts glutamic acid into the neurotransmitter gamma-amino-butyric-acid (GABA). GABA is a neuroinhibitory transmitter that regulates many aspects of brain function. Around one third of all the nerve cells in the brain send inhibitory, rather than accelerating, signals, and this is done via GABA.

Taking L-glutamine increases the production of GABA. This process can also be aided synergistically by taking 50 milligrams of vitamin B6 daily. Increased levels of GABA in the brain serve as a natural calming and memory-enhancing agent, and generally help one to think more clearly. L-glutamine is also useful for people who tend to use alcohol to help them cope with stress, as it reduces the craving for alcohol.

The recommended dosage of L-glutamine is 500 milligrams, twice daily. L-glutamine should be taken on an empty stomach, preferably with fruit juice.

Royal Jelly

Royal jelly is a natural food supplement that is rich in many essential vitamins, minerals, enzymes, hormones, and amino acids. It also contains antibiotic components. Royal jelly has energy-boosting properties, making it useful for symptoms of fatigue as well as for improving memory and overall mental and physical functioning. (For further information about royal jelly, see Chapter 9).

Essential Fatty Acids

The health benefits of essential fatty acids are huge and diverse, and could be the subject of an entire book. Essential fatty acids (EFAs) are vital for the production and release of many hormones, including sex hormones and adrenal hormones. They are also an integral part of cell membranes, and they give these membranes the proper flexibility and suppleness. They stop your cells from drying out and give them normal cohesiveness.

There are two basic types of EFAs, known as omega-3 and omega-6. These nutrients can help overcome dry and/or itchy skin, dry hair, hair loss, dry eyes, and dry mouth, and can reduce vaginal dryness. They also help to reduce infections of the skin and mucous membranes such as cystitis, vaginitis, and mouth ulcers.

Many women use expensive creams and shampoos, to no avail; their skin and hair remain unhealthy. This is because they are lacking in EFAs. If you feed your skin and hair from within by using EFAs, you will be delighted with the difference—but give it time. It usually takes three to four months to see results.

Other benefits of EFAs include an improvement in the functioning of the nervous system, so I recommend them for women with a poor memory, insomnia, or mood disorders. Many women find that EFAs have the added benefit of reducing hot flashes, presumably because EFAs enhance and balance the production of sex hormones and prostaglandins. (For information about the role of EFAs in the production of prostaglandins, see Chapter 7). EFAs exert an anti-inflammatory effect and can reduce the pain of arthritis and general muscular aches and pains.

Essential fatty acids must be obtained from foods like fish, fish oils, and unprocessed fresh vegetables, seeds, nuts, and botanical oils. To boost your intake of omega-6 EFAs, take 2,000 to 3,000 milligrams of evening primrose oil, 1,000 milligrams of lecithin, and 1,000 milligrams of spirulina daily. To increase your level of omega-3 EFAs, take 1,000 to 2,000 milligrams of fish oil capsules daily or increase your consumption of fish to four servings weekly. In addition, use one tablespoon of cold-pressed canola, olive, or sunflower oil in your salad daily. Another tasty way to boost your levels of EFAs at breakfast time is to grind a mixture of flaxseeds, almonds, and sunflower seeds and sprinkle it on your cereal or rice (see page 115).

Herbs

There are many herbs that contain plant estrogens or that act to stimulate the production of your natural hormones. These herbs can "bridge the gap" between the time when your ovaries cease their estrogen-producing function and when your adrenal glands start producing a different form of estrogen, called estrone. Estrone is not as powerful as the estrogen produced by the ovaries, which is called estradiol; however, it is often enough to reduce unpleasant symptoms during this transition period.

Table 6.2 lists herbs that are suitable for use in menopause, with a brief overview of their actions, as well as information on how to use them. Herbs can be purchased from health food outlets or from a qualified herbalist.

The appropriate method of preparing an herbal remedy from fresh herbs depends on which part of the plant is used. The flowers and leaves of herbs may be prepared by making a tea. Bring water to a boil on top of the stove. While the water is boiling, place the herbs in a glass or ceramic (not metal) teapot that has a tight-fitting lid. Use one-half ounce (approximately one tablespoon) of the dried herb to one cup of water. When the water boils, pour it over the herbs, cover, and let the tea steep for ten to fifteen minutes. Then strain it and drink. You can sweeten the tea with a teaspoon of honey if needed.

If you are using the dried root, seeds, or woody parts of a plant, you will need to make what is called a decoction. Place one-half ounce (about one tablespoon) of the dried herb in a glass or enamel (not metal) saucepan and add one cup of cold water. Let the herbs soak in the water for ten minutes, then cover the pot and bring it to a boil over high heat. Reduce the heat and let the mixture simmer for fifteen

Table 6.2 Herbs for Menopause

There are many medicinal herbs that can be helpful for the menopausal woman. This table lists those herbs that I have found to be most valuable, together with their actions and uses. These herbs should be available through an herbalist or at better health food stores.

Herb	Part Used	Actions and Uses
Black cohosh (*Cimicifuga racemosa*)	Dried roots and rhizomes	This is a good estrogenic herb that acts specifically on the uterus to reduce cramps and congestion. It is also good for relieving hot flashes. Black cohosh contains two antirheumatic agents and it is an excellent herb for relieving muscular pain and cramping. It may also help to reduce cholesterol levels and blood pressure. Take 250 mg in tablet or capsule form, two to four times daily. Or take ½ teaspoon of tincture, twice daily.
Chaste tree (*Vitex agnus-castus*)	Dried fruit	This herb is a hormone balancer that is used to alleviate depression at menopause. Take 300–600 mg in tablet or capsule form daily. Or take ½ teaspoon of tincture, twice daily.
Damiana (*Turnera diffusa*)	Dried leaves	Damiana is a great herb for menopause because it is a pituitary regulator and antidepressant. It is also an aphrodisiac and is of benefit for sexual difficulties. It should not be taken too frequently, however, or it may irritate the lining of the urinary tract; I recommend taking 100–150 mg in tablet or capsule form, for two or three days out of the week. Or take ½ teaspoon of tincture, twice daily, for two or three days out of the week.
Dandelion (*Taraxacum officinale*)	Leaves, roots, and tops	Dandelion is a wonderful herb for the liver. If your hormones are out of balance, then your liver is under extra stress, and dandelion root will be beneficial for this. Take 1,000–3,000 mg in tablet or capsule form, or 2–3 cups of tea, daily. Or take 1–2 teaspoons of dandelion tincture, three times daily.

Herb	Part Used	Actions and Uses
Dong quai (*Angelica sinensis*)	Roots	This herb is high in natural plant estrogens called phytosterols and helps to reduce the symptoms of estrogen deficiency. Take 500 mg in tablet or capsule form, twice daily. Or take ½ teaspoon of tincture, twice daily.
False unicorn root (*Chamaelirium luteum*)	Dried roots and rhizomes	This plant is an estrogen regulator. It has a direct action on the uterus and ovaries and is considered to be a corrective herb for women. It is a specific for the herbal treatment of ovarian cysts. Take 500 mg in tablet or capsule form, or 1 teaspoon of tincture, daily.
Ginkgo (*Ginkgo biloba*)	Leaves	This herb improves brain function, circulation, and oxygenation of all body cells. It is helpful for symptoms of fatigue, memory problems, and depression. Take 1,000 mg in tablet or capsule form daily. Or take 1 teaspoon of tincture, twice daily.
Ginseng (*Eleutherococcus senticosus, Panax quinquefolius*)	Roots	Ginseng strengthens the adrenal glands, enhances immune function, increases energy, and normalizes blood pressure. It is useful for symptoms of both mental and physical fatigue. Take 1,000–4,000 mg in tablet or capsule form daily. Ginseng is a safe energy-booster for most people. However, if you have very high blood pressure (over 180/100), you should avoid it. Siberian ginseng appears to be more effective than the American variety.
Licorice (*Glycyrrhiza glabra*)	Dried roots and rhizomes	Licorice is a powerful adrenal stimulant and is a wonderful estrogenic herb. For this reason, it is a very useful herb during menopause. Care must be taken, however, not to take licorice too often, or it can deplete potassium and elevate blood pressure. If you have high blood pressure, use it with caution or avoid it entirely. On the other hand, if you suffer from low blood pressure, this herb will be useful in correcting the problem. Licorice makes a pleasant-tasting tea. It can also be added in small amounts to other herbal teas to improve their flavor. For hot flashes, I recommend drinking 1–2 cups of licorice tea or taking 500–1,000 mg in tablet or capsule form daily. Or take ½–1 teaspoon of tincture, twice daily.

Herb	Part Used	Actions and Uses
Liferoot (*Senecio aureas*)	Dried plant	Liferoot is a uterine tonic that contains plant estrogens. It helps to reestablish emotional and vascular stability and eliminate hot flashes. It may also help to treat irregular, painful, or excessive menstrual bleeding. Take 500 mg daily in tablet or capsule form. Or take ½ teaspoon of tincture, twice daily.
Raspberry (*Rubus idaeus*)	Fresh or dried leaves and fruit	Raspberry is an astringent and nutritive estrogenic herb. It has a direct action on the muscles of the uterus, helps to tone weakened uterine muscles, and relaxes uterine and intestinal spasms. It also assists in correcting prolapse of the uterus and/or vagina. Take 2,000 mg in tablet or capsule form, or drink 2–3 glasses of raspberry tea daily. Or take ½–1 teaspoon of raspberry tincture, up to three times daily.
Red clover (*Trifolium pratense*)	Dried flower heads; fresh plant	Red clover contains a plant estrogen called coumestrol and one of its medicinal actions is to stimulate the ovaries. It is a good "alkalinizing" herb that is described in herbals as an *alterative,* which means that it restores healthy body functions. Red clover is a specific for the herbal treatment of ovarian cysts. To relieve hot flashes, take 1,000–2,000 mg of red clover in tablet or capsule form or drink 3–4 cups of red clover tea daily. Or take ½–1½ teaspoons of red clover tincture, up to three times daily.
Sage (*Salvia officinalis*)	Fresh or dried leaves	This herb has many medicinal properties and is very useful during menopause for the treatment of hot flashes. Sage reduces excessive sweating and it contains plant estrogens. You will find sage particularly helpful in eliminating night sweats. Drink 3–4 cups of sage tea daily to relieve hot flashes, or take ½–1 teaspoon of tincture, three times a day. Sprinkle finely chopped fresh sage in soups and on salads and vegetables.
St. Johnswort (*Hypericum perforatum*)	Fresh or dried flowering plant	This herb is a mild sedative that is specific for anxiety states. It may also be useful for combatting depression. Take 500 mg in tablet or capsule form, or ¼–1 teaspoon of tincture, two or three times daily.

Herb	Part Used	Actions and Uses
Sarsaparilla (*Smilax officinalis*)	Dried roots and rhizomes	Sarsaparilla is another alterative herb that stimulates the production of testosterone and therefore improves a flagging libido. It also helps to increase energy. Take 1,000–2,000 mg in tablet or capsule form or drink 2–3 glasses of sarsaparilla tea daily. Or take ¼–½ teaspoon of tincture, up to three times daily.
Saw palmetto (*Serenoa serrulata*)	Dried fruit	This herb is an astringent diuretic that is beneficial for the treatment of urinary incontinence, fluid retention, and prolapse of the pelvic organs. Dryness and lack of tone in the tissues of the bladder often lead to irritation and weakness. This is reduced by saw palmetto. This herb can also be useful for combatting chronic urinary tract infection. Take 1,000–2,000 mg in tablet or capsule form daily. Or take ½ teaspoon of tincture, twice daily.
Shepherd's purse (*Capsella bursa-pastoris*)	Dried flowering plant; fresh plant	Shepherd's purse is a pituitary regulator with androgenic properties. One of its primary attributes is its ability to normalize progesterone levels. If you are moving into menopause and have been experiencing excessive, irregular bleeding or spotting, this herb will help to regulate and increase the length of your menstrual cycles until the natural cessation of menses. Take 500 mg in tablet or capsule form daily, or take ¼–½ teaspoon of tincture, up to twice daily.
True unicorn root (*Aletris farinosa*)	Dried roots and rhizomes	This estrogenic herb stimulates and strengthens the female genital organs. It is a bitter herb that is also useful for indigestion and has a mild sedative action. Take 500–1,000 mg in tablet or capsule form daily. Or take ½ teaspoon of tincture, twice a day.
Wild yam (*Dioscarea villosa*)	Dried roots and rhizomes	Wild yam is a powerful estrogenic herb used by women around the world. It has a good anti-inflammatory action and gives relief from menopausal arthritis. It also has progestogenic properties, and may help to reduce heavy menstrual bleeding. Take 1,000–4,000 mg of dried extract daily. Or take ½ teaspoon of tincture, twice a day.

minutes. Then remove the pot from the heat and let the mixture steep for another ten minutes. Strain it and drink it warm.

Whether you are using a tea or a decoction, I recommend that a cupful be taken warm, not hot, three times a day.

If you do not have the time or inclination to prepare your own herbal teas, you may take herbs in dried form as tablets or capsules. Herbs are also available in the form of tinctures, which are liquid extracts, and as dried extracts, which can be turned into tablets and capsules. Both tinctures and dried extracts are concentrated sources of herbs, so smaller amounts are required to achieve the same effect. In general, I recommend that herbs be taken in tea, tablet, or capsule form, rather than as tinctures, because tinctures contain varying concentrations of the active ingredient, they tend to be very strong-tasting, and they contain alcohol. Consult a qualified herbalist, an herb shop, or your local health food store for availability and for good, reputable brands of herbs.

STRATEGIES FOR HEALTHY BLOOD VESSELS

Naturopathic medicine is useful not only for treating the acute discomforts of the perimenopausal period, but also has a role to play in preventing or reducing some of the health problems that result from the lack of estrogen over the long term. As discussed in Chapter 2, after menopause, women are at significant risk of heart and blood vessel disease. Indeed, cardiovascular disease is the number-one killer of women in Western societies, claiming twice as many lives every year as cancer. Although these diseases tend to attack women later then men, this should not stop women from looking for ways to decrease their risk. Furthermore, the survival rate for women who suffer heart attacks is lower than that for men, regardless of age.

Let us take a look at some of the nutritional strategies you can use to decrease your risk of cardiovascular disease. These good nutritional habits will also reduce your risk of cancer and obesity.

Minimize Fats

Reducing the amount of fat in your diet will lower your risk of heart disease and cancer. Fats and oils are extremely high in calories, and if you eat excessive amounts of them, they slow down your metabolic rate, keeping you from losing weight and contributing to obesity.

Much of the fat in your diet can be eliminated simply by changing your habits and cooking techniques. One basic principle that will help to cut the amount of fat in your diet is to cut down on meat and dairy products and to increase the proportion of your diet that consists of grains, legumes, fruits, and vegetables. This will also take a load off your kidneys and help you retain calcium. Another way to lessen the amount of fat in your diet is to stop buying processed foods such as packaged cookies, cakes, pastries, and fried foods, which are high in fat.

Avoid frying your foods (especially deep-frying!) and roasting or baking meats in their own fat. Broiling, boiling, steaming, and dry-baking are better. The one exception to this rule is stir-frying, which can be done with a minimum of added oil in a non-stick, non-aluminum pan. When you must use oil, use small amounts of cold-pressed vegetable oils such as canola, olive, sunflower, or grapeseed, and cook your food slowly, at lower temperatures, to avoid having the oil become oxidized. Resist the temptation to add salt or use prepackaged sauces; instead, flavor your foods with vegetable extracts, tomato purée, herbs, and spices.

When you select a prepared food product such as breakfast cereal, take the time to read the product information on the packaging. You may be surprised to find that some popular brands have very high levels of fat, salt, and sugar. Good low-fat alternatives to processed breakfast cereals are oatmeal and natural, unsweetened muesli, as well as barley and brown rice, which can be boiled and eaten as a hot cereal with the addition of a little low-fat milk.

You can also make an excellent mixture called LSA (for *l*inseeds-*s*unflower seeds-*a*lmonds) that can be added to your breakfast cereal. Mix 1½ cups of linseeds (flaxseeds), 1 cup of sunflower seeds, and ½ cup of almonds together and grind them into a fine meal in a food processor or grinder. LSA is an excellent concentrated source of omega-6 essential fatty acids, fiber, natural plant estrogens, protein, calcium, selenium, vitamin E, vitamin A, and the B vitamins. It must be kept fresh; store it in the refrigerator. Start making healthy choices and feel the benefits.

Saturated Fats

When reducing the amount of fat in your diet, it is important to know that all fat is *not* created equal. In particular, saturated fats are the most important ones to eliminate, as consuming excessive amounts of them can lead to obesity, clogged arteries, and an increased risk of cancer of the breast, ovaries, uterus, and bowel. The most identifiable feature of saturated fats is that they are solid at room temperature.

Examples of saturated fats are the fats found in beef, pork, lamb, poultry, cheese, chocolate, butter, copha, suet, and lard. Meat drippings, whole milk, cream, ice cream, and coconut and palm oils also contain saturated fats. I am not saying that you must avoid these foods completely, but you should keep your consumption of them to as low a level as possible. Make sure that you remove all the fat from meat and the skin from chicken, and use low-fat dairy products. You may eat as much as two to three servings of red meat per week, provided you remove all the fat. Never fry red meat or chicken; bake or broil these meats or use them in casseroles and stews.

Eggs may be eaten in moderation, up to four per week. Eggs contain cholesterol, but they also are an excellent source of the sulfur-containing amino acids L-cysteine and L-methionine. L-cysteine contains a form of sulfur that inactivates free radicals and thus protects and preserves cells. It is also a precursor of glutathione, which is a major antioxidant in the body. L-methionine helps to eliminate fatty substances that can otherwise clog the blood vessels, and it is vital for efficient liver function, which helps to rid the body of toxins. The sulfur-containing amino acids found in eggs can thus be considered anti-aging foods. Always boil or poach your eggs, rather than frying them; when fried, eggs produce oxycholesterol, or oxidized cholesterol, a dangerous fat that generates free radical production in the body.

Processed or delicatessen meats, such as processed luncheon meats, smoked or pressed ham, salami, and pepperoni, are not healthy to eat, as they are loaded with saturated fats. Moreover, because they are not fresh, their fats may become rancid. Rancid fats are highly oxidized and generate free radicals in the body that attack blood vessels and body cells. Also, these meat products contain nitrites, which have been linked to the development of cancer.

Cholesterol

Cholesterol is a pearly fatlike substance that is produced in your liver. It cannot dissolve in water or blood, so it is transported in the bloodstream by specialized molecules called lipoproteins. Lipoproteins are not found in foods, but are manufactured by the liver, and they come in two basic types: high-density lipoproteins (HDL) and low-density lipoproteins (LDL). HDLs are scavengers that pick up free cholesterol in the blood and carry it back to the liver to be reused or broken down. LDLs are larger than HDLs and are heavily laden with cholesterol, which they transport to the body's cells, as needed.

Cholesterol is actually a necessary substance, and if you do not eat any foods that contain it, your body will make it. It becomes a problem, however, when there is more of it present than your body can cope with. Thus, if your diet contains a lot of cholesterol, it may end up being deposited on the walls of your arteries, leading to hardening and blockage of the arteries. To prevent this, it is necessary to have enough HDL circulating in your bloodstream to scavenge excess cholesterol and prevent it from causing harm. You can increase your levels of beneficial high-density lipoproteins by exercising regularly, reducing the amount of saturated fats in your diet, maintaining a healthy weight, and not smoking.

Your body can produce all the cholesterol you need without the need for added dietary cholesterol. If you consume very little dietary cholesterol, your need for high-density lipoproteins will also be low. Generally, it is ideal to have a cholesterol level of less than 200 milligrams per deciliter of blood (200 mg/dL). In some people, elevated blood cholesterol may increase the risk of heart disease. Cholesterol is found mostly in foods of animal origin, such as meat, poultry, seafood, eggs, and dairy products. However, it is not only the amount of cholesterol but also the amount of saturated fats in the diet that affects a person's blood cholesterol level. This is because, when excessive amounts of saturated fats are eaten, the body responds by converting the fat into cholesterol. Foods high in saturated fats include all land animal products such as fatty meats, preserved meats, and whole-milk dairy foods; other sources are shellfish and coconut and palm oils.

Reducing dietary saturated fat is very important, but it is only one of the methods of reducing cholesterol levels. You must also increase your consumption of foods that help to lower cholesterol. These include oily fish (such as salmon, sardines, and tuna), vitamin-C-rich foods (citrus fruits, melons, cabbage, fresh green leafy vegetables, kiwi fruit, sweet and chili peppers, and strawberries), garlic, onions, and foods containing soluble fiber. Soluble fiber is fiber that dissolves easily in water and is found in the gums, pectin, and mucilages of plant fiber. Good sources of soluble fiber are legumes, cereals, whole grains, oat bran, fruits, and vegetables. Soluble fiber protects against gallstones, ulcerative colitis, high blood pressure, high blood cholesterol, and diabetes.

Unsaturated Fats

Unsaturated fats are fats that are liquid at room temperature. Examples are fish oils and olive, flaxseed, canola, grape seed, peanut, corn, safflower, sesame, soybean, and sunflower oils. These oils are combinations of monounsaturated and polyunsaturated oils. The best choices among these oils are olive, canola, and flaxseed. This is because these oils contain large amounts of monounsaturated oils. Research has shown that these oils can be beneficial to the health of our arteries.[3] Mediterranean peoples have consumed these oils regularly for centuries, and have very low rates of heart disease.

Try to obtain cold-pressed vegetable and seed oils, as no fat or oil is healthy if it is subjected to heat processing or if food is fried in it. Both animal fats and vegetable oils, when they are heated to high temperatures, form chemicals that attack and destroy blood vessel walls.

If you use butter or margarine, do so only in moderation (if you are trying to lose weight, it is best to avoid these products altogether). Butter is a natural product, but it is high in cholesterol, saturated fat, and calories. Margarine is a synthetic product that is made by subjecting vegetable oils to a process called hydrogenation. This is what makes margarines solid or semisolid at room temperature. However, hydrogenation also results in the creation of substances called cis- and trans-fatty acids. Cis- and trans-fatty acids are not useful nutritional substances and, if consumed regularly in large amounts, can have negative effects on your cardiovascular system. In addition, many brands of margarine contain other added chemicals to make them look and taste more like butter. Thus, while some people once thought that margarine was a healthy alternative to butter, it is now known that a small amount of butter is probably better for you than any amount of margarine. I recommend that you use a spread like tahini, avocado, or hummus instead of either margarine or butter.

Cut Down on Salt

Salt is a compound of two elements, sodium and chloride. Standard table salt consists of 40 percent sodium and 60 percent chloride. Our nutritional requirement for sodium is only 250 to 350 milligrams each day. One level teaspoon of salt contains 2,000 milligrams of sodium, so it is easy to see that many of us eat too much salt. Excess salt in the diet increases your risk of developing high blood pressure, cardiovascular disease, fluid retention, and osteoporosis.

Many menopausal women consume too much sodium. This is not surprising when you consider how much salt is added to processed and convenience foods, and that the salt and pepper shakers are standard additions to the dinner table.

Table 6.3 Percentages of Fatty Acids in Different Oils

Oils from vegetables, seeds, and nuts contain different mixtures of saturated, monounsaturated, and polyunsaturated fats. It is the chemical structure of a fatty acid that determines which class it belongs to. The consumption of saturated fats tends to raise cholesterol levels and has been linked to obesity, heart disease, and a number of different types of cancer. On the other hand, oils high in monounsaturated fatty acids, such as olive, canola, and avocado oil, are beneficial in that they can lower total cholesterol levels. Polyunsaturated fats are sources of essential fatty acids. This table illustrates the relative proportions of the types of fatty acids found in commonly used oils.

Oil	Percentage of Saturated Fatty Acids	Percentage of Mono- unsaturated Fatty Acids	Percentage of Poly- unsaturated Fatty Acids
Avocado	10.0	70.0	10.0
Canola	6.0	60.0	34.0
Coconut	92.0	6.0	2.0
Flaxseed (linseed)	6.0	24.0	70.0
Grape seed	11.1	17.3	71.6
Olive	10.0	82.0	8.0
Safflower	8.0	13.0	79.0
Sesame	13.0	46.0	41.0
Sunflower	8.0	26.0	66.0

There are several things you should do to reduce your sodium intake. Read labels on processed foods and avoid products that contain salt or sodium in any form. Watch for "hidden" sodium, in the form of flavor enhancers and preservatives, such as monosodium glutamate (MSG), hydrolyzed proteins, autolyzed yeast, sodium caseinate, and calcium caseinate. Occasionally, MSG is included in salt shakers at fast food outlets or used to add a different flavor to French fries or chicken; it is a well-known addition to Chinese food. Other label terms that may indicate the presence of sodium in processed foods include malt flavoring, high-flavored yeast, yeast extract, soybean extract, textured soy protein, and even such harmless-sounding terms as "spices" or "seasonings." Artificial sweeteners can also contain high levels of sodium. Reducing your intake of processed and fast foods usually leads to a large reduction of dietary sodium levels.

Finally, stop adding salt to your cooking and put away the salt shaker! At first you will miss the salty taste. You may have strong cravings for salt for even the first few months, but they will pass. Eventually, your taste buds will readjust and you will be able to taste the more subtle natural flavors of foods again.

Nutritional Supplements for a Healthy Heart

Vitamin A, vitamin C, vitamin E, beta-carotene, and choline, and the minerals zinc and selenium, are known as the antioxidant nutrients. They help to reduce damage to the blood vessels caused by free radicals. (For information about free radicals and antioxidants, see Chapter 7). If possible, find a good-quality antioxidant tablet containing all of these nutrients. If not, you can take each component separately. I recommend that you take the following daily:

- 10,000 international units of vitamin A *or* 20 milligrams of beta-carotene.
- 4,000 milligrams of vitamin C with bioflavonoids.
- 100 to 500 international units of vitamin E.
- 30 milligrams of zinc chelate.
- 500 milligrams of choline.
- 50 micrograms of selenium.

Vitamin E is required for energy production and enables muscle cells to use oxygen (the fuel for energy) more efficiently. It is thus beneficial for athletic people and for those wanting to reduce symptoms of heart disease, such as angina and palpitations. Vitamin E reduces oxidant damage to LDL cholesterol and the blood vessel walls, thereby helping to keep your arteries unclogged and your blood flowing freely.

A study conducted at Boston's Brigham and Women's Hospital and the Harvard School of Public Health showed that daily supplementation with vitamin E in doses of 100 to 400 international units reduced the risk of heart attack by 25 to 50 percent in both men and women.

Garlic is the most popular food herb in the world today. It contains compounds such as sulfur-containing amino acids, antioxidants, selenium, and allicin, which exert beneficial effects on the blood vessels and the immune system. It acts as a natural body cleanser and antibiotic. Best of all, it reduces levels of LDL (the so-called "bad cholesterol") and reduces the tendency to form blood clots. You may eat garlic fresh or cooked in food, or take odorless garlic capsules; 1,000 to 2,000 milligrams (one to two grams) daily is a suitable dose.

Magnesium is a mineral that is vital for heart muscle relaxation and that improves metabolic function and energy production in the heart muscle and blood vessel walls.[4] Good dietary sources of magnesium are wheat germ, nuts, soybeans, legumes, whole grains, all dark-green vegetables, and milk. You can also take magnesium tablets. Recommended doses are 400 to 800 milligrams daily.

The herbs ginkgo biloba and bilberry contain bioflavonoids that have a vitamin-C-like action and strengthen the capillaries (tiny blood vessels) in your cardiovascular system. They are available in tablet or capsule form at pharmacies and health food stores. You can take from 1,000 to 2,000 milligrams of ginkgo biloba and up to 1,000 milligrams of bilberry daily. The supplement coenzyme Q_{10} also plays an important role in energy production in the heart, brain, and body muscles. I recommend a daily dose of 100 to 200 milligrams.

FOODS FOR HEALTHY BONES

Osteoporosis, one of the most serious long-term consequences of estrogen deficiency, is common among postmenopausal women, but it is not inevitable. Good nutrition, especially the consumption of adequate amounts of calcium and other minerals, has an important part to play in both preventing and in slowing the progression of this disease.

Generally speaking, for healthy bones, women require 800 to 1,000 milligrams of calcium daily. During pregnancy, lactation, and menopause, calcium needs increase to 1,000 to 1,500 milligrams daily.

Good food sources of calcium include dairy products, salmon, tuna, sardines (with the bones), green leafy vegetables, and tofu. Table 6.4 lists foods that are good sources of calcium. Use it to see if your daily diet provides you with an adequate amount of calcium. If your diet falls short of this, or if you are not sure, take a good-quality calcium tablet to give you 1,000 milligrams of calcium daily.

One of the best food sources of calcium is milk. A cup of milk daily will give you a good start to meeting your calcium requirements. When it comes to cow's milk, I recommend calcium-enriched milk, such as Borden's Hi-Calcium or Viva with extra calcium, which is low in fat and much higher in calcium than skim milk. If you are on a dairy-free diet, you may choose calcium-enriched soy milk instead. Some soy milks are calcium enriched, while others are low in calcium, so read labels to be sure the product you choose is a good source of calcium.

There are a number of different supplemental sources of calcium. Bone meal, which comes from the ground bones of young animals, contains calcium from microcrystalline hydroxyapatite. Bone meal calcium is well absorbed, but it is possible for it to be contaminated with heavy metals such as lead. Calcium carbonate, which contains 40 percent elemental calcium, is the most concentrated and cheapest form, but its absorption varies. Calcium lactate, calcium citrate, and calcium gluconate are less concentrated forms of calcium (containing around 15 percent elemental calcium) but are better absorbed than the carbonate forms.

Some calcium supplements contain a mixture of different types of calcium to improve absorption. Many good calcium supplements also contain vitamin D (cholecalciferol), which enhances the absorption of calcium from the intestines. Calcium is best absorbed when taken on an empty stomach, although if need be it can be taken with food. It should *not*, however, be taken with high-fiber foods such as cereals, grains, and legumes, as this will reduce its absorption. It can be taken with dairy products, fruits, vegetables, or meats.

To test the absorbability of a calcium supplement, place it in vinegar at room temperature for half an hour, stirring it every few minutes. After this time, the supplement should be completely dissolved. If it isn't, then it won't dissolve in your stomach, either, and you should switch to another brand that passes the vinegar test.

Our bones contain magnesium and the trace minerals zinc, silica, boron, and manganese in addition to calcium, and studies suggest that adequate amounts of all these different minerals (see pages 104–107) are more effective than calcium alone at preventing bone loss. If your diet is not always perfect, I suggest that you take a trace mineral tablet that contains all of these minerals. Calcium and other mineral tablets are best taken last thing at night before going to bed.

In addition to making sure you obtain sufficient calcium and other minerals in your diet, avoid making dietary mistakes that can steal minerals from your bones. Keep your consumption of protein from animal sources (meat, fish, dairy products) to no more than 50 grams daily. This is the equivalent of the amount of protein found in a six-ounce serving of meat or fish plus one eight-ounce glass of milk.

Table 6.4 Food Sources of Calcium

Many different foods contain calcium, but some contain more than others. This table will give you an idea of which foods are the best sources of calcium. Use it to see whether your normal diet is providing you with the recommended 1,000 milligrams of calcium per day. If not, you should either include more calcium-rich foods in your your diet or take supplemental calcium to make sure you get enough of this vital mineral.

Food	Serving Size	Milligrams of Calcium
DAIRY PRODUCTS		
Buttermilk	1 cup	285
Cheese		
American	1 ounce	174
Camembert	1 ounce	110
Cheddar	1 ounce	204
cottage	1 cup	135
cream	1 ounce	23
feta	1 ounce	140
Monterey jack	1 ounce	212
mozzarella, part-skim	1 ounce	207
Muenster	1 ounce	203
Parmesan, grated	1 tablespoon	69
ricotta, part-skim	½ cup	335
Swiss	1 ounce	219
Cow's milk		
low-fat (2-percent)	1 cup	297
skim	1 cup	302
skim, powdered	1 tablespoon	130
whole	1 cup	291
Egg	1 large	25
Goat's milk	1 cup	350
Half-and-half	1 tablespoon	16
Sour cream	1 tablespoon	16
Yogurt, plain		
whole-milk	1 cup	275
nonfat-milk	1 cup	452

Food	Serving Size	Milligrams of Calcium
FISH		
Clams, canned	3 ounces	78
Crabmeat, canned	3 ounces	38
Flounder or sole, baked	3 ounces	16
Haddock, broiled	3 ounces	51
Oysters, Eastern, raw	1 cup	111
Salmon, pink, canned	3 ounces	181
Sardines, canned, drained	3 ounces	325
Shrimp or scallops, cooked	3 ounces	39
Tuna, light, canned	3 ounces	10
NUTS AND SEEDS		
Almonds, unsalted	1 ounce (about 25 nuts)	70
Brazil nuts, unsalted	1 ounce (7–8 nuts)	55
Pistachio nuts (unsalted)	1 ounce (about 23 nuts)	40
Sesame seeds, ground (if seeds are not ground, calcium is unavailable)	1 ounce	290
Sunflower seeds	1 ounce	30
Walnuts, unsalted	1 ounce (about 25 nuts)	30
Tahini	1 tablespoon	85
LEGUMES AND SOY PRODUCTS		
Baked beans	½ cup	60
Chickpeas	½ cup	75
Hummus	1 tablespoon	15
Kidney beans	½ cup	60
Lima beans	½ cup	40
Miso	½ cup	92
Peanut butter	1 tablespoon	6
Peanuts, roasted	½ cup	54
Refried beans, canned	½ cup	59

Food	Serving Size	Milligrams of Calcium
LEGUMES AND SOY PRODUCTS, continued		
Soy milk	1 cup	10
Soy milk, calcium-enriched	1 cup	40
Soybeans, cooked	½ cup	90
Tofu	½ cup	130
FRUITS		
Apple	1 medium	10
Apricots, dried, uncooked	1 cup	100
Avocado	1 medium	26
Banana	1 medium	7
Blackberries, raw	1 cup	46
Blueberries, fresh, raw	1 cup	9
Cantaloupe	½ medium	29
Dates, whole, pitted	10 medium	27
Figs, dried	10 medium	269
Grapefruit	½ medium	14
Grapes, seedless	10 medium	5
Kiwi fruit	1 medium	20
Mango	1 medium	21
Orange	1 medium	30
Papaya	1 medium	72
Peach	1 medium	4
Pear	1 medium	20
Pineapple, fresh, cubed	1 cup	11
Prunes, uncooked	10 medium	43
Raspberries	1 cup	27
Rhubarb, cooked	½ cup	170
Strawberries	1 cup	27
Watermelon	4-inch wedge	30
VEGETABLES		
Asparagus, fresh, cooked	½ cup	22
Beets, cooked	½ cup	15
Bok choy, fresh, raw	½ cup	37
Broccoli, fresh, cooked	1 medium spear	83

Food	Serving Size	Milligrams of Calcium
VEGETABLES, continued		
Brussels sprouts, fresh, cooked	½ cup	28
Cabbage		
cooked, drained	1 cup	50
raw	1 cup	32
Carrot		
fresh, cooked	½ cup	24
fresh, raw	1 medium	19
Cauliflower, fresh, cooked	½ cup	17
Celery, fresh, raw	1 medium stalk	16
Collard greens, cooked	½ cup	27
Green beans, fresh, cooked	½ cup	29
Kale, fresh, cooked	½ cup	47
Mustard greens, cooked	½ cup	76
Okra, fresh, cooked	½ cup	50
Onions		
cooked	½ cup	23
raw	1 medium	30
Peas, green, cooked	½ cup	19
Potato, baked, with skin	1 medium	20
Pumpkin, canned	1 cup	64
Spinach		
cooked, drained	½ cup	130
raw, fresh	½ cup	27
Squash, acorn or butternut, mashed	½ cup	52
Sweet potato, cooked	1 medium	32
Turnip, cooked	½ cup	18
Zucchini, cooked	½ cup	12
GRAINS AND GRAIN PRODUCTS		
Barley, cooked	1 cup	17
Bread, most types	1 slice	30
Breakfast cereal, most types	1 cup	5–30
Bulgur, cooked	1 cup	18

Food	Serving Size	Milligrams of Calcium
GRAINS AND GRAIN PRODUCTS, continued		
Farina, cooked	1 cup	147
Granola, homemade	1 cup	76
Oatmeal, cooked	1 cup	19
Pasta, enriched, cooked	1 cup	10
Rice, brown, cooked	1 cup	20
Rice, white enriched, cooked	1 cup	23
MISCELLANEOUS		
Basil, ground	1 teaspoon	32
Celery seed	1 teaspoon	38
Chocolate, milk, plain	1 ounce	50
Cinnamon	1 teaspoon	28
Molasses		
blackstrap	1 tablespoon	137
light	1 tablespoon	33
Sugar, brown	1 tablespoon	12

Avoid foods that contain phosphorus or phosphate additives. These include many processed foods and fizzy soft drinks. If you consume beverages containing alcohol or caffeine, either eliminate these items from your diet or keep your consumption to a moderate or low level. (For further information on dietary risk factors for osteoporosis, see Chapter 2.)

As a doctor who has treated menopausal women for twenty years, I have seen my attitudes change and evolve over time. In my early days, I believed that hormone replacement therapy was the crucial factor in helping women to cope with menopausal problems and improve their health. In later years, I came to see the vital importance of nutrition and natural medicine. By using specific nutritional supplements and reducing the amount of fat, salt, refined sugars, and chemical additives in your diet, you provide a much stronger foundation for long-lasting health, youthfulness, and vitality than HRT alone could ever provide. The re-energizing power of nutritional and herbal medicine will never cease to amaze you once you learn to use its tools.

Chapter 7

SLOWING DOWN
THE AGING PROCESS

As a doctor, I find that a significant percentage of women are worried that the onset of menopause signals a sudden increase in their rate of aging and that their looks will fade overnight. But this need not occur, if you learn how to reduce some of the things that tend to accelerate the aging process.

The rate at which you age is determined by several factors. The ones you cannot control are your genetic inheritance and the age at which you pass through menopause. Factors over which you *can* exert control include exercise, diet, lifestyle, exposure to the sun's ultraviolet rays, and the health of your immune system.

EXERCISE

Exercise is vital for women in midlife. After menopause, the body's metabolic rate decreases, causing a tendency to gain weight easily. Fifty percent of postmenopausal women experience an increase in body weight of at least ten pounds, and in many cases much more. Ideally, you should do at least twenty to thirty minutes of aerobic exercise daily to stimulate your heart, blood circulation, and respiration. This can consist of doing aerobic exercise to music (at a gym or in your own home), swimming, doing aqua-aerobics, jogging, or working out on a stationary bicycle or stair-climbing machine.

If you have not done any aerobic exercise before, the process should be started gradually. Begin with five minutes a day and gradually increase the amount of exercise over a four-week period, until you reach thirty minutes daily. If you smoke or if you have any cardiovascular risk factors, such as obesity, high blood cholesterol levels, diabetes, high blood pressure, or a family history of heart

disease, you should have a full fitness checkup, including a cardiac
stress test, done by a medical doctor before you undertake any aerobic
exercise. If you have arthritic joints or a back problem, doing aerobics,
jogging, and strenuous weight-bearing exercise may aggravate pain
and damage. In that case, modified yoga, tai chi, swimming, and
walking would be excellent choices, as they stretch the joints gradually and keep the muscles in tone.

Many menopausal women find that aerobic exercise can be awk-
ward because of stress incontinence. This means that when pressure
in the abdomen is temporarily increased by exercise (or by straining,
sneezing, coughing, etc.), urine is passed uncontrollably, soiling the
underclothes. This often happens in menopause because a deficiency
of estrogen can cause the pelvic floor muscles to weaken and sag so
that the bladder is not sufficiently supported. Exercises to strengthen
the pelvic floor muscles can overcome stress incontinence in 40 to 50
percent of cases (see Chapter 8).

EXPOSURE TO THE SUN

As far as aging of the skin is concerned, there is nothing worse than
the ultraviolet (UV) radiation from the sun. Of course, protection from
this radiation should begin at a young age, but many women who are
now menopausal were not taught about the harmful effects of the sun
while they were growing up, so it is common to see sun-damaged skin
in this age group.

There are two different types of ultraviolet rays, UVA and UVB
rays. UVB rays are stronger in the middle of the day and in the
summer, and are the major cause of sunburn and skin cancer. UVA
rays are present regardless of the season and time of day, and
although they do not usually cause sunburn, they do contribute to
skin cancer and premature aging, particularly with long-term exposure.

To protect yourself from the sun, whenever you are outdoors, use
a sunscreen cream or lotion with a sun protection factor (SPF) of at
least 15. If you are very fair skinned, red-haired, blonde, or blue-eyed,
you will be safer choosing an SPF higher than 15. Whatever SPF you
choose, look for products that specify *full spectrum protection*. This
means that they screen out both UVA and UVB rays. Apply the
sunscreen to all exposed areas of skin every two hours—more often
if you are swimming or perspiring a lot. Avoid spending time outdoors between 10:00 A.M. and 3:00 P.M., when UVB rays are strongest,

without good protection. In addition to sunscreen, wear a broad-brimmed hat and protective clothing, making sure to protect your neck and face, as these areas really show your age. Use good-quality sunglasses that specify broad-spectrum UV protection to filter out the ultraviolet rays.

THE ANTI-AGING DIET

A woman in midlife need not be fanatical about diet, as obsessions can cause an early death through stress or boredom. However, there are four basic principles that should be followed for profound and far-reaching benefits to your physical and mental well-being. These principles are:

1. Learn to love *raw* vegetables and fruits. Ideally, around 50 percent of your diet should consist of raw foods. Raw foods are living foods, and by virtue of this they stimulate the metabolism and aid in the elimination of toxic waste materials from the body. Raw foods contain beneficial molecules such as antioxidants and indoles, which have anticancer properties and are excellent for overcoming obesity, arthritis, and high blood pressure.

   Ideally, a woman in midlife should buy herself a juice-extracting machine with which to make raw vegetable and fruit juices on a daily basis. Juices not only supply essential minerals and vitamins, but also contain easily assimilated organic compounds such as vegetable amino acids, which improve digestion, have natural antibiotic properties, and promote healthy intestinal flora. This reduces bad breath. Raw fruit and vegetable juices are distinct and incomparable in their rejuvenating and regenerating effect on the human organism. No other source supplies as much vitamin C as fresh fruits and vegetables do, and this vitamin is entirely destroyed when the juices are subjected to heat.

   Generally, a pint of juice daily is the smallest amount that will yield worthwhile results. If you can manage more, so much the better; one quart may be needed to stimulate a quicker process of detoxification and rejuvenation.

   Recommended juices include:

   • A combination of two or more of the following: apple, grapefruit, orange, strawberry, pear, pineapple, and peach.

   • A combination of two or more of the following: carrot, celery, tomato, parsley, cucumber, cabbage, spinach, beet, radish, dandelion, lettuce, turnip green, and watercress.

For a health cocktail, add a dash of lemon, strawberry, and honey to either of the above recipes.

2. Avoid chemically processed and frozen foods, and buy foods in their natural state. Fresh foods in their natural state contain less bacteria than processed frozen foods and thus promote healthy intestinal flora and good digestion, and reduce bad breath. Natural foods also contain more fiber, vitamins, and minerals; fewer calories; and less fat. Choose unprocessed grains, cereals, seeds, nuts, legumes, and whole-grain bread instead of products made with white flour, sugar, sweeteners, colorings, salt, commercial sauces, and hydrogenated oils. In addition to lacking any nutritional value, many artificial food additives are suspected of causing health problems ranging from allergies to headaches to cancer. Refined sugar and its various relatives (such as brown sugar and corn syrup) add little to the diet except calories. Furthermore, they cause your blood sugar level to rise very rapidly, and then to fall again just as rapidly. Such wild fluctuations in blood sugar can lead to lethargy and headaches, as well as aggravating many unpleasant menopausal symptoms.

3. Reduce your intake of fats. This means reducing not just cholesterol, but all fats, especially saturated fats. Avoid fatty meats such as lamb, pork, ham, bacon, chicken with the skin, and processed meats, as well as fried foods, coconut, processed margarines, and whole-milk dairy products. You should especially avoid fats that have turned rancid. Oils that have been subjected to very high temperatures (repeated deep-frying, for example) and oils that are not fresh are likely to become rancid. Rancidity leads to the production of free radicals, which increase inflammation and promote the development of cancer (see page 133). Substitute monounsaturated and polyunsaturated fats for saturated fats by eating foods such as broiled fish, canned fish, tahini, hummus, seeds, grains, legumes, almonds, vegetables, and cold-pressed vegetable and seed oils.

4. Drink eight to twelve glasses of water daily. The best type of water is pure bottled water or water that has passed through a reverse-osmosis filter system attached to your kitchen tap. If you live in an area that is generally free of air pollution, pure rainwater is an option as well. Water dilutes the blood, thereby reducing cholesterol and acidity and improving sluggish circu-

lation. It helps to flush toxins from all of the body's tissues, reducing your body's exposure to these substances. It also improves kidney function and lowers blood pressure.

ANTIOXIDANTS

To understand the process of aging, it is essential that you know about *free radicals*. These sound like political terrorists, and indeed they are dangerous, unstable electronic particles that terrorize our cells. They rush around the body damaging cell walls, genetic material, blood vessel walls, joints, and intracellular components. When free radicals are produced in your skin, they damage the collagen, a protein that is an essential component of skin tissue and is responsible for the skin's elasticity. Free-radical damage causes cross-linkage and degeneration of collagen fibers, resulting in wrinkling, thinning, and aging of the skin. These evil free radicals cause an atomic-bomb-type chain reaction in our precious cells that keeps on generating more and more free radicals. Obviously, we all hate free radicals, as they damage our cells, leading to more rapid aging. All of us would like to reduce the production of free radicals in our bodies.

To some degree, free radicals are inevitable. They are formed when we are exposed to polluted air, cigarette smoke, rancid dietary fats, some highly processed chemical foods, fluorescent lights, video display units, viruses, and alcohol, among other things. But there is still a great deal we can do to protect our cells against their destructive effects.

Antioxidants are substances that scavenge and neutralize free radicals. They act as a defense system for our cells. Because they prevent and reduce cell damage, they help to prevent degenerative diseases and to slow down the aging process. There are a number of different kinds of substances that act as antioxidants, including vitamins, minerals, enzymes, and amino acids. Some of the most potent are vitamins A, C, and E, and choline; the amino acids methionine and cysteine; and the mineral selenium. Many of these, you will notice, are the same nutrients that are recommended for easing the acute symptoms of menopause (see Chapter 6), so they really offer dual benefits.

Vitamin E

One of the best ways to protect our tender tissues from free radical damage is to take vitamin E supplements. Vitamin E was the first recognized antioxidant. It has been known for many years for its anti-aging effects, since long before scientists knew of the existence or understood the significance of free radicals.

One word of caution, however: Only natural forms of vitamin E are useful. Unfortunately, thousands of women erroneously take synthetic forms of vitamin E, which are of negligible use. The natural forms of vitamin E are called dextro-tocopherols (or d-tocopherols). These d-tocopherols are a mixture of alpha, beta, gamma, delta, eta, epsilon, and zeta tocopherols (different variants of natural vitamin E that have slightly different chemical configurations), and they all play valuable roles in scavenging and neutralizing free radicals. D-alpha-tocopherol is the most common natural form of vitamin E sold in supplement form. Synthetic vitamin E is denoted by d*l*-alpha-tocopherol. The natural forms of vitamin E are 30 percent more active (that is, effective) as antioxidants. Doses of 500 to 1,000 international units of vitamin E a day can help to slow down the aging process. Vitamin E is also present in fresh wheat germ, nuts, and eggs, and in cold-pressed vegetable oils such as soybean, olive, sunflower, sesame, and safflower oil.

According to Dr. Jeffrey Blumberg, a cancer specialist at Tufts University in Boston, the incidence of cancer could be cut in half if people increased their consumption of antioxidants by making dietary changes and taking nutritional supplements. Vitamin E can inhibit the development of cancer of the skin, breast, and colon. Dr. Blumberg has found compelling evidence that you can add years to a healthy life by taking sufficient antioxidants. He recommends taking supplements of vitamins A, C, and E, or eating between five and nine servings of fresh vegetables each day.

Beta-Carotene and Vitamin A

Another free-radical fighter is the nutritional substance called beta-carotene, which is found in high concentration in certain vegetables, such as carrots, beet greens, sweet potatoes, and pumpkin. That is one of the reasons why raw vegetable juices are so wonderfully good for age-conscious folks. If you consume too much beta-carotene, your skin may turn a slightly yellow or bronze color, as carotene is a yellow pigment. This is harmless and is not equivalent to vitamin A overdosage. If it happens, simply reduce your intake of beta-carotene until the bronze color fades.

It is possible to take beta-carotene in supplement form. A dose of 5,000 international units (six milligrams) can safely be taken one to three times daily. Beta-carotene is converted in the liver into vitamin

A, which is beneficial because vitamin A is itself a powerful free-radical scavenger and so a useful anti-aging substance. It is especially important for the strength and metabolism of the skin and mucous membranes, which are particularly vulnerable to drying and infection in menopausal women. As an alternative to beta-carotene, daily doses of 5,000 to 10,000 international units of vitamin A are generally helpful and safe. However, if you suffer from any medical disorders, check with your doctor first before taking vitamin A.

Vitamin C

The miraculous anti-aging and rejuvenating properties of vitamin C are to the water-soluble parts of your body (such as intracellular fluid and serum) what vitamin E is to the fatty parts (such as cell membranes). Vitamin C is a powerful antioxidant and free-radical scavenger and is extremely important in maintaining the integrity of the collagen in your skin and bones, and thus the elasticity of these tissues. Vitamin C reduces the rate of aging of the skin and bones.

The best sources of vitamin C are fresh fruits and vegetables, but as a nutritional "insurance policy," I recommend that all women take a daily supplement of 1,000 to 2,000 milligrams of vitamin C in the form of calcium ascorbate, which is easily dissolved in raw fruit and vegetable juices. Calcium ascorbate is nonacidic and so is better for people who find the ascorbic acid form of vitamin C too acidic, and it is the best type of vitamin C supplement for menopausal women because it also provides some calcium. Some people become hypersensitive or allergic to vitamin C supplements, even esterified vitamin C ("Ester-C"), which is normally well tolerated. If this happens to you, make sure you eat plenty of foods high in vitamin C, such as fresh raw fruits and vegetables.

According to Dr. Judie Walton, a gerontologist at the Aging Research Institute at Concord Hospital in Sydney, Australia, vitamins E and C are known to prolong life in experimental animals, and she expects that the same will be shown to be true for humans. Dr. Walton says that this is logical as, if the antioxidant vitamins protect specialized cells (such as those of the brain, heart, liver, lungs, blood, and immune system), these cells will not need to be replenished so often from our cell banks. The cell banks are stores of undifferentiated (primitive) cells found in the bone marrow, spleen, liver, and blood. These primitive cells are used to replace dead cells throughout the body. If body cells do not need to be replenished as often, the cell banks should thus last longer and the individual's life span should increase accordingly.

Selenium

Selenium is an essential trace mineral that is essential for optimal health. It is also an important antioxidant. The body uses selenium to produce an intracellular antioxidant enzyme called glutathione peroxidase. This enzyme reduces oxidant damage to cell membranes, to the nucleic acids DNA and RNA, and to cell proteins, and thus is an ally in the fight against aging. Adequate selenium is vital for this enzyme to function effectively. Selenium can provide useful protection against cancers, especially breast cancer, and a large range of degenerative diseases.

The best food sources of selenium are brewer's yeast, garlic, mushrooms, celery, onions, radishes, fish, grains, broccoli, cabbage, cucumbers, and organ meats, although the potency of these foods as sources of selenium may vary tremendously, depending on soil conditions in the places where they were produced. Selenium can be taken in supplement form, as inorganic sodium selenite, or in organic form in the foods mentioned above or in a special brewer's yeast enriched with selenium. Organic forms are probably preferable. Daily doses range from 50 to 200 micrograms of selenium.

ESSENTIAL FATTY ACIDS

Essential fatty acids (EFAs) are components of unsaturated fats that are necessary for health and vitality. They are termed *essential* for two reasons:

1. Our bodies are unable to manufacture them.
2. Our cells cannot function normally without them.

If a patient of mine asks me what the most important supplement is for health and beauty, I respond, "Essential fatty acids." This is because the membranes that surround and protect each cell in the body are made of essential fatty acids (see Figure 7.1). The physical integrity and energy production of our cells depends upon adequate amounts of essential fatty acids (EFAs) in the diet.

If our cell membranes break down or weaken, they may no longer be able to prevent dangerous particles (toxic chemicals, infectious

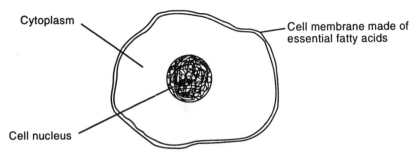

Figure 7.1 A Body Cell

organisms, viruses, and free radicals, among others) from passing through them. If such dangerous particles manage to pass through a weakened cell membrane, they enter the "inner sanctum" of the cell, where they may inflict severe damage. Such damage may be irreparable and result in physical, chemical, and electrical impairment of the cell. If cellular damage is widespread, it can result in chronic inflammation and degeneration, as well as increasing the rate of aging of the cells. If a cell's nucleus, which contains the genetic control center of the cell, is severely damaged, the cell may be transformed into a cancer cell. So you can understand why it is vital to have strong, healthy membranes around your cells to protect them. This is one of the most important strategies for slowing down the aging process and enabling us to look, feel, and act younger longer.

Essential fatty acids are the most important nutrients for building and maintaining strong and efficient cell membranes. The antioxidants—vitamins A, C, and E, beta-carotene, and selenium—also help our cell membranes to keep out nasty invaders like free radicals and viruses. To use an analogy, one might think of a body cell as a castle. The cell membrane is the moat and brick wall around the castle; antioxidants are the defending army, shooting arrows from the parapets to weaken and repel the castle's invaders.

There are two types, or families, of beneficial EFAs: omega-6 and omega-3. Omega-6 EFAs are linoleic and gamma-linolenic acids. Omega-3 EFAs are alpha-linolenic and eicosapentaenoic acids.

EFAs not only strengthen cell membranes, but they also help to optimize the balance between vitally important hormonelike chemicals called prostaglandins. There are three families of prostaglandins: prostaglandin 1, prostaglandin 2, and prostaglandin 3. Let's call them PG_1, PG_2, and PG_3.

The PG_1 and PG_3 families are beneficial to the body because they reduce inflammation and regulate the function of many hormonal glands and also the brain's chemistry. As outlined in Table 7.1, omega-6 EFAs are used by the cells to produce PG$_1$ and omega-3 EFAs are used to produce PG$_3$. The production of beneficial PG$_1$ and PG$_3$ is desirable and promotes a healthy immune system. In particular, PG$_1$ acts as a powerful messenger in the body and increases the production and release of many different hormones, including thyroid hormone, cortisone, growth hormone, and sex hormones, as well as of neurotransmitters (brain chemicals that transmit messages from one nerve cell to another). Thus, omega-6 EFAs, by increasing PG$_1$, keep your hormonal glands and brain cells "switched on." Because of this, a woman with mental fatigue, emotional imbalances, chronic fatigue syndrome, or adrenal gland exhaustion should take omega-6 EFAs to boost her PG$_1$ levels.

Where can you obtain EFAs? They can be found in certain foods (such as fish, grains, beans, and seed oils) as well as in nutritional supplements. The best way of increasing your intake of EFAs is to take daily supplements of evening primrose oil (2,000 to 4,000 milligrams), flaxseed meal (two tablespoons of ground seeds), black currant seed oil (1,000 milligrams), and/or fish oil (1,000 milligrams). Also, include fresh and canned fish, seeds, vegetables, and cold-pressed seed oils in your diet regularly. EFAs are vulnerable to damage from high temperatures, light, air, or hydrogenation, which makes them unusable by the body. In particular, the body cannot transform damaged EFAs into prostaglandins. That is why the best oils are those that are extracted from their source using a cold-pressed or expeller-pressed process, and that are not refined with chemicals, bleaches, solvents, or deodorants. Seeds or olives that are passed through a screw press, for example, release their oils without having to be subjected to high temperatures. Oils that are not filtered excessively retain more source nutrients.

Hydrogenated margarines, fried foods, and commercially processed oils all contain damaged fats. Many commercial cookies, pastries, cakes, crackers, and cereals also contain unhealthy fats, such as highly saturated palm and coconut oils, hydrogenated vegetable shortening, and margarine. Avoid these unhealthy fats, and try to use only unrefined cold-pressed monounsaturated or polyunsaturated oils.

Increasing your intake of EFAs can help you in many ways:

• Improving the appearance and health of your skin, hair, and nails.
• Increasing your mental and physical energy.
• Boosting your immune system.

Table 7.1 Functions and Sources of Fatty Acids

This table provides an overview of selected fatty acids, together with the types of prostaglandins they are used to produce, the effects of these prostaglandins on the body, and food sources of the fatty acids. The correct balance of fatty acids—specifically, more omega-3 and omega-6 essential fatty acids and less arachidonic acid—is needed to create the optimal balance of prostaglandins in the body.

Prostaglandin Family Produced From These Fatty Acids	Actions of These Prostaglandins in the Body	Food Sources of These Fatty Acids
LINOLEIC ACID AND GAMMA-LINOLENIC ACID (OMEGA-6 ESSENTIAL FATTY ACIDS)		
PG_1 (desirable)	Reduce pain and inflammation; improve skin; increase energy and vitality.	Breast milk; sesame, safflower, cotton, and sunflower seeds and oil (cold-pressed); corn and corn oil; soybeans; raw nuts; legumes; leafy greens; black currant seeds and their oil; evening primrose oil; borage oil; gooseberry oil; spirulina; soybeans, lecithin.
ALPHA-LINOLENIC ACID AND EICOSAPENTAENOIC ACID (EPA) (OMEGA-3 ESSENTIAL FATTY ACIDS)		
PG_3 (desirable)	Reduce pain and inflammation; help circulation.	Fresh fish from cold, deep oceans (such as mackerel, tuna, herring, sablefish, flounder, sardines, salmon); rainbow trout; bass. Fish must not be fried. Also, flaxseed oil; black currant and pumpkin seeds and their oil; cod liver oil; shrimp; oysters; leafy greens; canola oil; soybeans; walnuts; wheat germ; wheat sprouts; fresh sea vegetables; fish oil capsules.
ARACHIDONIC ACID (AA) (OMEGA-6 *NON*ESSENTIAL FATTY ACID)		
PG_2 (undesirable)	Excess amounts may increase pain and inflammation and can result in excessively sticky blood platelets and poor circulation.	Animal meats; whole-milk dairy products; preserved meats; fried foods; processed and takeout foods; coconut and palm oils.

• Reducing inflammation and aches and pains.

• Improving your circulation and reducing your chance of developing cardiovascular disease (or, if you already suffer from cardiovascular disease, reducing its severity).

• Reducing cellular damage, thereby slowing the rate of aging and reducing your risk of developing cancer.

• Reducing breast pain and tenderness.

• Improving gynecological health by reducing menstrual cramps, ovarian cysts, and pelvic inflammation.

As you age, your body becomes less efficient at manufacturing PG_1 and PG_3, and this is partly why you may slow down and suffer increasing aches and pains with advancing years. Also, as you age—and especially if your diet is high in saturated fats—you produce increasing amounts of the undesirable PG_2 family of prostaglandins. PG_2 promotes the body's inflammatory response, so its action tends to increase inflammation and pain. You can reduce the amounts of undesirable PG_2 in your body by reducing your total fat (especially saturated fat) intake, maintaining normal body weight, not overeating, and ensuring adequate intake of omega-3 and omega-6 EFAs, the B vitamins, zinc, and vitamins C and E. Many menopausal and postmenopausal women complain of a variety of painful syndromes, such as headaches, arthritis, rheumatism, and backaches. This is largely due to an imbalance in prostaglandins—too much PG_2 and not enough PG_1 and PG_3. In such cases, doctors may prescribe anti-inflammatory drugs known as antiprostaglandins, such as naproxen (Naprosyn) and diclofenac sodium (Voltaren), to suppress the body's production of PG_2. These drugs work quickly and effectively to relieve pain and inflammation, but if taken for many months, they may cause unpleasant side effects.

If my patients complain of pain and inflammation in their muscles, bones, and joints, I prefer to teach them how to reduce these problems with nutritional medicine, rather than having them rely on anti-inflammatory drugs alone. And this is not hard to do. Simply:

• Reduce the amount of saturated fats in your diet.

• Increase the amount of omega-3 and omega-6 essential fatty acids in your diet (see Table 7.1).

• Take antioxidant supplements daily.

• Take vitamin B complex and zinc supplements at least twice weekly.

• Drink one to two quarts of water and at least one pint of raw vegetable juices daily.

The essential fatty acid story sounds too good to be true. However, I have recommended EFAs to thousands of women in poor health, and I can assure you that it is worthwhile to increase the amount of EFAs in your diet. As you grow older, you need to "oil"—but not to "grease"—to slow down the aging process.

If you would like to know more about research into EFAs, you can write to Stephen Wright, M.D., at the Royal Free Hospital, School of Medicine, London, England. Or refer to *Heal Cancer* by Ruth Cilento, M.D., and/or *Making Fats and Oils Work for You* by Lewis Harrison.[1]

BOOSTING YOUR IMMUNE SYSTEM

Your immune system is the surveillance and defense system that protects your cells against infections, toxins, free radicals, and damage from such factors as radiation exposure (including sun exposure), poor diet, stress, cancer, and exposure to chemicals. The immune system is very complex and involves the lymphatic system, liver, spleen, bone marrow, and thymus gland. The thymus gland, situated in the lower part of the back and behind the breastbone, or sternum, is the master gland of the immune system and orchestrates the activities of the other parts.

Unfortunately, the valuable thymus gland shrinks with age, leading to a general reduction in the efficiency of the immune system. As your aging immune system weakens, you become more susceptible to degeneration and inflammation of the cells, to infections, cancer, and even more rapid aging. All of these things combined may eventually shorten your life span.

Thus you can comprehend the huge importance of a healthy immune system in the quest for youthfulness and a longer life. The immune system acts to reduce damage and aging of the most vulnerable parts of our cells, such as the nuclei and intracellular metabolic structures.

There are many simple, commonsense measures you can take to promote the health of your immune system:

• Avoid exposure to tobacco smoke, both from smoking and from secondhand smoke.

• Avoid exposure to toxic chemicals such as pesticides and solvents.

• Avoid engaging in high-risk behavior such as intravenous drug use, unprotected sexual activity, and poor hygiene, all of which increase the risk of unnecessary infection.

• Avoid unnecessary surgery. Always get a second opinion before agreeing to any non-emergency surgical procedure.

• As much as possible, avoid stress. Steer clear of vexatious people and situations! Learn stress management techniques to help you cope with problems that are not avoidable.

• Keep the amount of fat in your diet to a minimum.

• If you drink alcoholic beverages, keep your consumption to a moderate level (no more than four to five drinks weekly).

• Avoid exposure to radiation, including excessive sun exposure and unnecessary x-ray or bone scan procedures. When using a computer, keep a distance of two and a half to three feet away from the screen, and four feet from the back and sides of the unit; when watching television, sit at least four feet from the set. If you use a microwave oven, check it periodically to make sure the door seals tightly, and step back at least six feet from it when it is on.

• Avoid excessive use of xenobiotic (nonorganic) drugs, especially painkillers, sedatives, and anti-inflammatory drugs.

• Avoid consuming foods that contain chemical preservatives, colorings, and flavorings, such as artificial sweeteners.

• Investigate your local environment. If possible, try not to make your home in an area that is highly polluted or located near such potential hazards as power generators or coal mines.

• Maintain a body weight appropriate for your height and build.

• Eat plenty of raw fruits and vegetables, whole grains, and legumes.

• Take antioxidant supplements (see page 133).

• Make sure to get an adequate amount of sleep, at least six to eight hours a night for most people.

• Get regular exercise (see page 129).

• Make time for relaxation and pleasurable activities on a regular basis.

• Drink plenty of water and fresh juices, a total of two quarts a day.

• Be yourself. Don't be afraid to assert your needs and talk about your feelings. Repressed emotions can increase the stress on your immune system.

If you take these simple measures to boost your immune system, you will likely be rewarded with a healthier, happier life, and quite possibly a longer one.

ANTI-AGING HORMONES

The body produces a number of natural hormones, such as growth hormone, thyroid hormone, and sex hormones, that help to keep us younger. They do this by maintaining muscular and skeletal mass, cardiovascular function, metabolism, and general function.

Growth Hormone

One powerful hormone involved in the aging process is growth hormone, which is produced by the pituitary gland. In the normal course of life, growth hormone production starts to decrease at about age twenty, and it continues to decline thereafter, reaching very low levels in some people by age sixty. This is usually accompanied by a reduction in muscle mass, metabolic rate, muscle strength, and exercise performance, and an increase in blood cholesterol level. Normal aging is growth hormone related. A deficiency of growth hormone causes fatigue; an increase in body fat, especially around the stomach; a slight reduction in muscle mass; cold hands and feet; a tendency to feel cold; and sometimes sexual dysfunction. Growth hormone deficiency affects men and women in equal numbers.

There is no question that people with abnormally low levels of growth hormone should receive treatment. Recently, American scientists obtained excellent results from giving injections of growth hormone to a group of healthy but growth-hormone-deficient men. In a study reported by Drs. Daniel Rudman, Axel Feller, and their coworkers in *The New England Journal of Medicine*, twenty-one healthy men from sixty-one to eighty-one years of age with low levels of growth hormone were studied.[2] They were representative of the approximately one third of all men in that age category who have subnormal levels of growth hormone. Twelve of the men were given injections of growth hormone for six months, and nine received no treatment.

The injections of growth hormone produced significant increases in lean body mass, spinal bone density, and skin thickness, with decreases in adipose (fat) tissue mass. In the nine men not on any growth hormone treatment, there were no significant changes. Six months of treatment with human growth hormone had an effect on lean body mass and adipose tissue mass that was equivalent in magnitude to the changes that normally take place in the course of ten to twenty years of aging.

The conclusion of the study was that diminished secretion of growth hormone is responsible in part for the decrease of lean body mass, the expansion of adipose tissue mass, and the thinning of the skin that occur in old age. This concept is supported by beneficial results of growth hormone treatment in growth-hormone-deficient adults. We know that injections of growth hormone can increase lean body tissue, muscle mass, and exercise performance, while reducing body fat and blood cholesterol. Still, questions about costs, benefits, safety, and side effects must be critically examined before growth hormone can be considered for general use in aging populations.[3]

You will be happy to know, however, that regular exercise seems to promote the production of growth hormone by the pituitary gland. Simply by exercising regularly, you can slow down the aging process by increasing your own supply of precious growth hormone in a natural way.

The Thymus Gland

Exciting new research in Europe and the United States shows that injections of extracts from the thymus gland may increase the resistance of the immune system to all diseases in animals. When these injections have been used in human beings, they have often produced a feeling of rejuvenation in the recipients. Further research could very well reveal that taking extracts of thymus will slow down the aging of the immune system.

The Thyroid Gland

It is not uncommon for the thyroid gland to become slightly underactive at the time of menopause. Indeed, women are far more prone to thyroid disease than men are. The thyroid gland controls the metabolic rate, and if it becomes underactive, the metabolic rate will decline, causing easy weight gain, difficulty in losing weight, dryness and thickening of the skin, dryness and thinning of the hair, constipation, sensitivity to cold, and mental slowness.

The functioning of your thyroid gland can be checked by a simple blood test. If your thyroid is found to be underactive, you will most likely be prescribed thyroid hormone, which will reestablish your metabolic rate and cause a return to normal body weight and mental activity. If your metabolism is a little sluggish and you seem to have trouble burning up the calories, yet your blood test shows that your thyroid gland is functioning within normal limits, you may be able to stimulate your metabolism by taking spirulina (a nutritional supplement) and macrobiotic dried seaweed preparations. These contain the essential mineral iodine along with other minerals that generally stimulate the metabolism.

The subject of aging is a fascinating one. Although we have made huge advances in understanding the factors that accelerate aging, we still cannot prevent it; we can merely slow it down. Still, this is a formidable achievement in itself. I hope that you will utilize the suggestions in this chapter about diet, exercise, nutritional supplements, and measures to boost your immune system to add both years to your life and life to your years. Life's main problem is, after all, its brevity. Even if we manage to avoid such hazards as nuclear war, poisonous spiders, and dull people, our biblical lot still totals only around 620,000 hours. This does not even give us the satisfaction of being "hour millionaires." Every hour is precious, and anything that we can do to add a few extra is well worth our effort.

Chapter 8

SEX AND MENOPAUSE

My patient Julie had had a hysterectomy for fibroids at the age of forty-seven. Two years later, she came to see me about her sex life, which was in total disarray. Julie related that for twelve months, she had not felt any sexual urges, and that when she had sex, it was merely to please her husband, who by all accounts was as virile as ever. During sex, Julie found that she experienced a burning pain and tightness in her vagina, which caused her to feel anxious and sweat profusely. Doctors use the term *dyspareunia* to describe painful sexual intercourse, and Julie's symptoms certainly fit into this category. Julie also complained that stimulation of her clitoris was no longer pleasurable; indeed, she had noticed that her clitoris was shrinking and felt tender and fragile.

"I'm definitely not the sexpot I used to be," Julie said, adding that she felt her husband was taking her lack of response personally, so that he was beginning to doubt his ability to be a passionate lover.

Examination of Julie's vagina showed it to be affected by a lack of sex hormones—it was pale in color and its mucous membranes were thin, dry, and fragile. Her clitoris was very small, inflamed, and tender. Thankfully, her ovaries felt normal and she had no sign of prolapse of the vagina. A blood test revealed that Julie had started menopause, as her levels of estrogen and testosterone were very low.

Julie decided that she wanted to try hormone replacement therapy to bring her hormonal levels back into the normal range. I reassured her that HRT would reverse the aging changes that had occurred in the sexual areas of her anatomy.

I gave Julie an injection of a mixture of natural estrogen and testosterone called Depo-Testadiol, which restores the levels of the sex hormones estrogen and testosterone in the body. Four weeks later Julie returned, saying, as I knew she would, that she had found her former sexual persona and was now able to enjoy sex, lubricate after stimulation, and have satisfying orgasms. Her dyspareunia had vanished. She was also pleased that the estrogen in the injection had made her shrinking breasts rounder and fuller.

Many women find menopause to be a sexually fulfilling and exciting time because they are better able to relax once they are free of the fear of unwanted pregnancy. They also tend to be more in touch with and comfortable about their sexual needs and desires than they were earlier in life. Unfortunately, however, there are also many women—like Julie—who find that menopause has an unfavorable impact on their sex lives. There are a number of different changes that can occur during menopause that may cause sexual problems.

VAGINAL DRYNESS

Many of the sexual difficulties menopausal women experience are a direct result of declining levels of sex hormones. Among other things, deficiencies of the sex hormones estrogen and testosterone often produce shrinkage and dryness of the vagina and vaginal lips (see Figure 8.1) and reduce sexual desire.

As discussed in Chapter 1, over half of all women at menopause and beyond are bothered by dryness of the vaginal tissues. This can lead to discomfort and even pain during sexual intercourse.

There are several different strategies that you can use, either singly or in combination, to overcome vaginal dryness and fragility. For a temporary lubricating action, you can use a bland jelly, such as K-Y jelly, or vitamin E cream, which also has a healing effect. These can be used before or during sexual intercourse, as needed. There are also products, such as Replens, that are formulated specifically for this condition and that, when used on an ongoing basis, are supposed to afford longer lasting relief. All of these products are available at drug stores without a prescription.

To actually restore and strengthen the vagina and vulva, however, you need to use a hormonal cream or vaginal suppositories, especially if your menopause was early or you want to resume sexual activity after a long period of abstinence. Hormonal creams and vaginal suppositories rejuvenate, thicken, and moisten the mucosal folds and lining of the vagina and the vaginal lips, and they improve blood circulation to the clitoral area, thus restoring the capacity for natural lubrication and orgasm. If you feel that your vagina has shrunk and is too small for your partner's penis, this can be overcome by regularly massaging the inside and opening of the vaginal walls using an estrogen cream. Place some estrogen cream on your fingers and rub

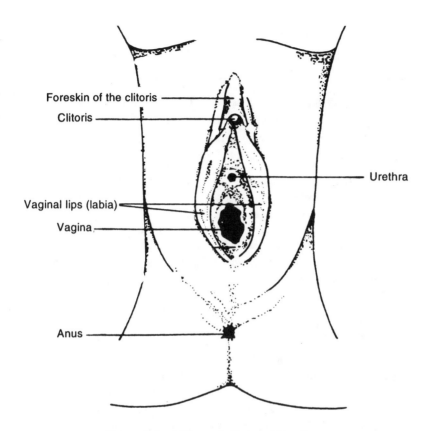

Foreskin of the clitoris

Clitoris

Urethra

Vaginal lips (labia)

Vagina

Anus

Figure 8.1 A Woman's External Sex Organs

it into the vaginal walls, gently stretching the walls apart and exerting gentle pressure backwards at the opening of the vagina. It is most comfortable to do this while lying down. It can be done gradually more and more each day. There is no need to stretch excessively and cause any discomfort. Ten minutes daily of this gentle massage and stretching is sufficient. Estrogen creams and suppositories require a doctor's prescription, as they contain hormones; suitable brands are Premarin, Ogen, and Estrace. For some women, especially if the clitoris has become very small, the addition of testosterone to the vaginal estrogen cream can make it much more effective than estrogen cream alone in restoring sexual responsiveness. The clitoris is normally the size of an average pea (see Figure 8.1).

You can ask your doctor to write a prescription for your pharmacist to mix you a special vaginal cream containing both estrogen and testosterone. While the precise proportions of ingredients may vary somewhat depending on the individual's needs, a good basic formula is as follows:

• 40 percent estrogen cream (Premarin cream or the equivalent).

• 20 percent testosterone (from ampoules of injectable Depo-Testosterone containing 100 milligrams per milliliter).

• 20 percent petroleum jelly.

• 20 percent Sorbolene and glycerine (made by mixing nine parts Sorbolene cream to one part glycerine).

You may massage your vagina, vulva, and clitoris with this cream every night for three to four weeks, after which time you should need to use it only twice a week. Some of my patients have told me that their hormonal creams or suppositories act like an aphrodisiac and make them feel more sexy!

POOR SEX DRIVE

If you are worried by a lack of sex drive, ask your doctor to do a blood test to measure your levels of the various hormones that are important determinants of libido and sexual well-being. It does not matter if you are already taking HRT, as some women on HRT still find that their sex lives are poor. This could mean that your HRT needs adjusting.

The blood test should measure four things:

1. Follicle-stimulating hormone (FSH). If your FSH level is very high, say, above 50 milli-international units per milliliter (mIU/mL), then you should benefit from taking estrogen (see page 7). If you already take estrogen, it may help to increase the dosage.

2. Estradiol. This is the biochemical name for estrogen. If the level of estradiol in your blood is consistently less than 54.4 picograms per milliliter (pg/mL), you may benefit from taking estrogen; if you are already taking HRT, a larger dose or different form of estrogen may help. If a woman taking estrogen tablets has a very active liver, it may break down the estrogen as soon as it is absorbed from the intestine and passes through the liver. In other words, the liver may weaken the effect of the estrogen before it

has a chance to work on your mind and sexual organs. If this is the case, you may find that you need increasing doses of estrogen tablets to feel normal, and yet your blood estrogen levels remain low. Increasing your dose of oral estrogen may help, but, of course, one cannot go on increasing the dosage of estrogen tablets indefinitely, as side effects such as nausea, fluid retention, and breast swelling may result.

If your liver is very active and your estrogen tablets are no longer relieving your symptoms, I suggest you ask your doctor about forms of estrogen that bypass the liver—namely, patches or injections—or that you take your estrogen tablets vaginally. Some women find that they get better results if they insert their estrogen tablets high into the vagina instead of taking them by mouth, because this allows the estrogen to be absorbed directly into the bloodstream from the vagina and thus bypass the liver. Consequently, some women find that their libido and sexual responsiveness improve after transferring to a form of estrogen replacement therapy that is not taken by mouth.

3. Sex hormone binding globulin (SHBG). This is a protein produced by the liver, and its function is to bind sex hormones such as estrogen, progesterone, and testosterone and carry them around in the bloodstream. In much the same way that a car transports you along a freeway, SHBG transports your sex hormones through your blood vessels. While they are bound to SHBG, however, the sex hormones are not active in your body. Thus, if you have too much sex hormone binding globulin in your blood, the majority of your sex hormones will be bound and inactive. Chances are that, as a result, you will feel not only sexless but tired and grumpy as well. On the other hand, if you have too little SHBG, this can result in acne or excess facial hair. Ideally, your SHBG level should fall somewhere in the middle of the normal range, which is 2700 to 8100 nanograms per milliliter (ng/mL). In other words, it is undesirable to have either too little or too much SHBG.

I see many women who complain of having lost their sexuality, and in many cases I find that their blood tests reveal very high levels of SHBG. Why is this? Once again, you can blame the liver, and it is the oral forms of estrogen that most stimulate the liver to produce increased amounts of SHBG. If your SHBG is high (8100 ng/mL or more), you may find that your sex life and general energy level improve if you transfer to a non-oral form of estrogen such as patches or injections, or if you take your estrogen tablets via your vagina. If the estrogen bypasses your liver in this way, the liver will be less stimulated to make SHBG and your levels of SHBG should start to fall.

If you have high levels of SHBG, a small dose of testosterone may also help as—don't forget—SHBG also binds the hormone testosterone, inactivating it. Testosterone is best given in the form of injections, and can really bring the zing back into a tired sex life.

4. Androgens. These are also sometimes referred to as "male hormones," but in fact women too require some of these masculinizing hormones in their bodies (albeit much less than men) to give them a healthy sex drive and to maintain general mental and physical well-being. The tests that are useful are those that measure total testosterone, free testosterone, and free androgens. The free hormones are the ones that are not bound by SHBG and thus are active in your body. If your doctor finds that your free testosterone and free androgen levels are very low, this can explain symptoms of fatigue and loss of sex drive, and these problems can easily be overcome by taking some testosterone in the form of injections.

Testosterone has the effect of increasing libido and may cause slight enlargement of the clitoris, depending on the dosage taken. Some women choose to take testosterone as part of their long-term program of HRT; others take it only initially or intermittently, say, once every four to six months. On the other hand, many women feel they do not need it at all. Your needs may change as you age, and your HRT can be modified to respond to this.

Poor libido can also be helped greatly by improving your diet and lifestyle. Avoid smoking and drinking excessive amounts of alcohol. Both of these can cause fatigue and reduce sexual response and performance.

The estrogenic foods mentioned in Chapter 6 can increase your estrogen levels naturally, so eat plenty of these during times of a sexual low. Soybeans, soy sprouts, and alfalfa sprouts, if eaten four to five times per week, will boost estrogen levels so that you may start feeling quite sexy again! The best herbs for increasing sex drive are damiana, dong quai, sarsparilla, red clover, and black cohosh (see pages 110–113). Also, take 2,000 to 3,000 milligrams of evening primrose oil, 500 milligrams of vitamin E, and 30 milligrams of zinc chelate daily to aid your adrenal gland in producing sex hormones.

How are your dreams? Are they lacking in sexual content? If so, try a combination of 500 milligrams of choline, 500 milligrams of pantothenic acid (vitamin B5), and 100 milligrams of vitamin B6 (pyridoxine) daily. This will boost your levels of the neurotransmitters serotonin and acetylcholine, which are involved in libido and sexual response. I see many husbands urgently writing this little combination down during my seminars on menopause!

INFLAMMATION AND INFECTION OF PELVIC TISSUE

Some menopausal women suffer from recurrent vaginal and bladder inflammation and/or infections that make them feel very tender and itchy, and most unsexy. These things occur partly because your sexual tissues are more vulnerable to infections and trauma without hormones. Hormone replacement therapy and vaginal creams can take care of this. If your vagina and vulva remain tender and inflamed and you continue to suffer bladder infections, urinary frequency, and burning, you need to boost your immune system with diet and nutritional supplements. To boost your immune system, I recommend the following:

- Drink two quarts of purified or bottled water daily.
- Drink two to three glasses of raw vegetable juices daily.
- Avoid refined sugar, alcohol, caffeine, cigarettes, foods containing refined sugar, and yeast products (eat yeast-free bread).
- Eat plenty of raw vegetables and fruit.
- Take 3,000 milligrams of evening primrose oil daily.
- Take an antioxidant supplement containing vitamin A or beta-carotene, vitamin C, bioflavonoids, vitamin E, and selenium. Take a total of 10,000 international units of vitamin A (or 20 milligrams of beta-carotene), 5,000 milligrams of vitamin C with bioflavonoids, 500 international units of vitamin E, and 50 micrograms of selenium daily.
- Take 1,000 to 2,000 milligrams of garlic or odorless garlic capsules daily.
- Take *Lactobacillus acidophilus* capsules or powder, or eat acidophilus yogurt daily.

These simple and safe strategies are extremely effective for overcoming recurrent infections or inflammation in the vagina and bladder, although they may take several months to bring relief. They are certainly safer than taking frequent courses of antibiotic drugs, which in the long term only weaken your own immune system. Please see your doctor if symptoms persist.

POOR GENERAL HEALTH AND MEDICAL PROBLEMS

If you suffer from chronic fatigue, severe stress, or any recurrent painful condition, or if you feel generally unwell, you will probably have a reduced interest in sexual activity as a result. See Chapters 6 and 7 for valuable information to help you improve your general health. You should also discuss any chronic or recurring health problems, and their effects on your sex life, with your health care provider.

Women who smoke heavily often notice a big reduction in their sexual response as they age. This is because the phases of sexual excitement, lubrication, and orgasm are due to the congestion and swelling with blood of the erotic tissues in the clitoris, vulva, and vagina. Smoking damages the small blood vessels all over the body, including those in the vaginal area, so that they are less able to swell up with blood in response to sexual stimulation. Thus, your sexual response can be impaired by heavy smoking.

PRESCRIPTION MEDICATIONS

A wide range of drugs may affect sexual function, causing loss of libido, difficulty in becoming sexually aroused, and orgasmic dysfunction. The most common drugs that cause these symptoms are appetite suppressants, some muscle relaxants, some drugs used to treat epilepsy, some drugs to prevent headaches, some high blood pressure medications, some sedatives and antidepressant drugs, some anti-ulcer drugs, and anti-male hormone drugs. Make sure you talk to your doctor about this before you begin taking a new medication, as you may be upset to find your sexual ability and desire lessened by the medication. There may be suitable alternative products that will not have this effect. New forms of many older drugs that have fewer side effects and no adverse effects on libido are becoming available.

PROLAPSE

Menopausal women may develop certain physical problems that can cause their sex lives to deteriorate—namely, prolapse of the vagina, bladder, bowel, and/or uterus. The term *prolapse* means a loosening and falling down of tissues or organs due to stretching and the force of gravity with advancing years. Areas prone to prolapse include the uterus and the back wall of the vagina. The front wall of the vagina may also prolapse. If it does, the bladder often prolapses with it, forming a swelling that can be seen when you cough. This combined bladder and vaginal prolapse is called a *cystocele*. Women with a cystocele often have problems with stress incontinence, meaning that when they cough, strain, or run, they pass urine involuntarily. If the back wall of the vagina prolapses, the lower bowel (the rectum) often prolapses down into it, forming a swelling that may fill with feces, especially if you are constipated. This swelling is called a *rectocele*. (See Figure 8.2.)

If the uterus prolapses down into the vagina, a more solid swelling can be felt or seen, and in severe cases, the cervix protrudes outside of the vaginal opening. Women with uterine prolapse have usually had several children, or experienced difficult and prolonged labor.

It is easy to understand why with any type of prolapse, sexual intercourse may be uncomfortable and perhaps a little embarrassing. Also, with prolapse, the vaginal and pelvic floor muscles are stretched to such a degree that both the woman and her partner may find the vagina too big for either of them to feel very much during intercourse.

In moderate to severe cases of prolapse, a surgical vaginal repair is necessary. This can be done completely through incisions in the vagina. A vaginal repair will eliminate a cystocele or rectocele, reduce or cure stress incontinence, and make your vagina a normal snug size so that sexual intercourse once again becomes enjoyable.

If your uterus has prolapsed down into the vagina, you will probably have a dull, dragging discomfort in your pelvic and vaginal areas. Your doctor will probably offer you a choice of surgical treatments: either having your uterus removed (hysterectomy) or having the uterine ligaments repaired so that the uterus is no longer prolapsed. In most cases of uterine prolapse, the uterus can be removed through the vagina at the same time a vaginal repair (if needed) is done, and this has the advantage that no abdominal incisions are required. Your gynecologist should explain the various surgical techniques to you in full before you decide which is best for you.

In milder cases of vaginal prolapse, Kegel's exercises, done to strengthen muscles in the vagina and pelvic floor, are often effective. These can be done in two ways:

1. Tighten and squeeze your vagina and rectum by drawing your muscles inward and upward. Hold this position for five to ten seconds, then relax. Repeat the exercise as many times as possible, gradually working up to 100 to 200 repetitions each day. This exercise can be done anywhere—while driving, sitting on the train, watching television, etc.—and no one can see you doing it.

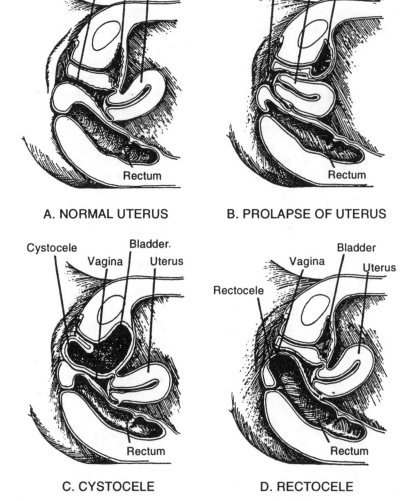

Figure 8.2   Different Types of Prolapse

After menopause, the ligaments and muscles that support a woman's reproductive organs in their normal position (figure A) can weaken. This can result in prolapse of the uterus (figure B), in which the uterus falls downward into the vagina, or of the vagina. If the front wall of the vagina prolapses, the bladder may prolapse with it, creating a cystocele (figure C). If the back wall of the vagina prolapses, the rectum may prolapse down into the vagina, forming a rectocele (figure D).

2. While passing urine, practice starting and stopping the flow of urine as many times as you can. This exercise will help women with stress incontinence.

If your prolapse is not too bad and you practice these exercises daily, after three to four months you may find that surgical repair is no longer needed. As an added bonus, you will find that your muscular control of the vagina and pelvic floor during sex has improved, thus giving greater sexual pleasure to both you and your partner.

YOUR STATE OF MIND

Some women find that menopause is a time of sexual liberation, and that their sex lives become better than ever. This may be because they no longer have to worry about pregnancy and contraception, and also because they have more time, space, and privacy to have a relaxed sex life. By the age of forty, most women have become aware of their sexual needs and preferences and feel comfortable about telling their partners how to please them. This is a wonderful thing, and very important for the sexual pleasure of both partners. If you find you are not able to fully express your sexual needs to your partner, it is very important that you try to improve communication. If you are not successful doing this on your own, it may be helpful to seek counseling.

Whether you are married or have an older or younger lover, menopause and the years surrounding it can bring you great sexual satisfaction. Many women tell me that their sex lives improve with age—"just like a good wine!" they say—and this is important to most women. So I want to reassure you that there *is* sex after menopause, and it can be very beautiful, gentle, and relaxing. The need to perform or be orgasmic mellows with age, and many couples find that sex becomes more emotional and affectionate.

On the other hand, if you would rather go to bed with a hot water bottle and a good book, that's normal, too. Many women find that once their sex hormones no longer surge, they feel a more intense urge to study, be creative, or take up new pursuits. For some women, it's great to no longer have men treating them as "sex objects," and they feel quite at ease saying, "Not tonight, darling, I've got to finish something else." The important thing is to enjoy being yourself, at both sexy times and tranquil times, during this unique phase of life.

Chapter 9

MALE MENOPAUSE— FACT OR FICTION?

This chapter is designed for both you and your partner, especially if he has a midlife crisis. We have all heard the phrase, whether used seriously or jokingly, but is there really such a thing as "male menopause"? In this chapter I will sort out the fact from the fiction. What you learn may surprise you.

The word *menopause* literally means the cessation of menstrual bleeding. In females, this signifies that the biological clock has stopped and infertility has set in, accompanied by dramatic hormonal changes. So technically, the word *menopause* obviously cannot apply to men. Yet it is indeed a fact that men also are vulnerable to fundamental emotional, mental, and physical changes at about fifty years of age and beyond.

HORMONAL CHANGES IN MEN

The production of testosterone by the testicles is at its peak during a man's twenties and thirties. Thereafter, a slow decline occurs. This decline becomes more noticeable after the age of fifty. However, there are large variations among individuals; some men at fifty produce such low levels of testosterone that they no longer feel any inclination to have a sex life, whereas others have high testosterone levels and are still sexually vigorous at eighty. As you read this, you are probably wondering how your partner (or you, if you are male) can be one of the lucky ones. The ability to produce testosterone is partly genetic, so in many cases it's "like father, like son." Lifestyle also plays a role. Men who smoke and/or who drink alcohol excessively have lower levels of testosterone in their blood than those who do not. Furthermore, as a man ages, not only does the production of testosterone diminish, but so does the ability of his tissues and cells to respond to testosterone.

Finding out if a man's testosterone level is down is a matter of a simple blood test. For men, the normal amount of testosterone in the blood is 290 to 1,420 nanograms per deciliter (ng/dL). A deficiency of testosterone is obvious if the blood level falls below 210 ng/dL. This would be further corroborated if the level of a pituitary hormone called luteinizing hormone (LH) is high, as this would indicate that the pituitary gland is trying to stimulate the sluggish testicles. This blood test may be repeated on three separate occasions, at eight-week intervals, to demonstrate a consistent deficiency of testosterone.

SYMPTOMS OF TESTOSTERONE DEFICIENCY

Testosterone deficiency shows up in a number of ways, including:

• Fatigue, reduced libido, and behavioral changes.

• Atrophy (shrinkage) of the muscles, testicles, and penis, and softening of the testicles.

• A reduced rate of growth of facial and body hair.

• A reduction in virility and the ability to achieve orgasm (in severe cases, impotence).

A man in midlife who previously had high levels of testosterone may find himself experiencing subtle mental and physical changes as a result of decreasing testosterone levels, even though blood tests reveal that his testosterone levels are still within the normal range. This is because even though technically normal, his testosterone level is much lower than it used to be, and he is sensitive to the decreasing level.

Subtle changes resulting from decreasing testosterone production may range from depression and loss of confidence to a loss of drive and a decline in aggression and competitiveness in all spheres. The warrior man may find himself becoming a bit of a mouse. If such a man gets himself to the doctor, he may be told that all this is symptomatic of a psychological midlife crisis, especially if a full checkup fails to reveal any medical problems. He may be told that this crisis is due to a plateau in his career, looming retirement, unrealized ambitions, getting older, stress, or just overdoing it. Consequently, he may be offered a course of antidepressants, sedatives, or tranquilizers, and referred for counselling to assuage his growing self-doubts. Men tend to be more reluctant than women to accept a course of such therapy;

many prefer to numb their anxieties at the bar with their buddies. Unfortunately, alcohol ingestion, if it becomes regular or excessive, often further reduces a man's production of testosterone, making his mental and physical imbalance worse.

It is vital to check the possibility of a hormonal contribution if a man in midlife experiences progressive symptoms of depression, loss of ambition, or loss of libido. And if tests suggest a deficiency of testosterone, hormone replacement therapy may be of help and a short course of testosterone replacement can be tried.

HORMONE REPLACEMENT THERAPY FOR MEN

The first semblance of HRT was actually used on a man, not a woman. In 1889, a then-famous neurophysiologist named Charles-Edward Brown-Sequard treated himself with an extract of animal testicles, which produced, in his own words, "a return of vigor, youthful appetites and desires." Today, hormone replacement therapy for men is available and can be taken in different forms, including oral androgens and androgen injections. Nowadays it is not unusual for a "menopausal" male to receive hormonal treatment, although the percentage of men who do is dramatically lower than the percentage of women who try HRT for menopause.

Oral Androgens

The word *androgen* is the medical term for the so-called male hormones—those sex hormones that have masculinizing effects on the body. Androgens may be taken on a regular basis in tablet form. Two common androgens available in tablet form are methyltestosterone (sold under the brand names Testred and Android) and fluoxymesterone (Halotestin). There is a possible link between methyltestosterone and liver cancer, however, and oral androgens can produce nausea if taken in large doses.

All in all, oral androgens are variable in their effect. Some men with severe testosterone deficiency complain that oral testosterone does not help them. In such cases, testosterone injections may be much more effective.

Androgen Injections

If a man is considering a short-term trial of HRT, there is probably no more definitive way of assessing its benefits than with a three- or four-month course of monthly injections of androgen. If a deficiency of testosterone is responsible for the mental, physical, and sexual fatigue of middle age, an androgen injection should greatly reduce, if not abolish, these symptoms within one to two weeks. This brings a great sense of relief. In addition to alleviating symptoms, androgen injections can produce a feeling of great energy and vitality, and can be a superb antidepressant.

Suitable injectable androgens are testosterone cypionate (found in Virilon and Depo-Testosterone) and testosterone enanthate (Delatestryl). Either of these can be taken as a deep intramuscular injection into the buttocks, usually once a month for three to four months. A follow-up appointment with the doctor should be made for three months after the final injection, by which time the effect of the injections should no longer be apparent. During this consultation, the decision either to abandon testosterone therapy or to continue with it for the long term can be made.

Side Effects of Androgen Replacement Therapy

If a man takes testosterone in any form—whether tablets or injections—on a long-term basis, the course of his therapy must be carefully supervised by a doctor. Testosterone replacement therapy taken over several to many years may cause side effects. The tablet forms are probably more likely to do this than are the other forms. Ideally, the lowest possible dose of testosterone that maintains a good quality of mental, physical, and sexual well-being should be used.

Testosterone replacement therapy can increase the size of the prostate gland. The prostate gland is a small, somewhat pyramid-shaped organ that is situated at the neck of the bladder and secretes fluid to add to the sperm during ejaculation. If the prostate gland becomes enlarged, a man may experience difficulty while passing urine, with such symptoms as difficulty in beginning urination, dribbling after passing urine, slowness and delay in completing urination, and urinary frequency. If these problems persist, surgical removal of the prostate gland may be required.

There are other potential consequences of testosterone replacement therapy as well. Long-term testosterone replacement therapy may increase the risk of cancer of the prostate gland. If testosterone doses are excessive, they may have an unfavorable effect on blood cholesterol patterns, increasing the risk of cardiovascular disease.

Excessive doses may also produce polycythemia (an abnormally high level of red blood cells) and significant weight gain.

Overall, however, testosterone replacement therapy—while not without risk—is safe and can be of tremendous value, provided it is prescribed by an expert in the field and followed up by annual checkups from a urologist.

CAN "MALE MENOPAUSE" CAUSE IMPOTENCE?

Minor degrees of testosterone deficiency do not cause impotence. A man's level of testosterone deficiency would need to be marked before inability to achieve erection and orgasm occurred. Most men who consult a doctor about impotence in midlife do *not* have a significant testosterone deficiency.

Other factors, such as general fitness, cardiovascular status, long-term abuse of cigarettes and alcohol, the consumption of certain medications, stress, and loss of confidence are more likely causes of impotence, especially if two or more of these factors occur in combination. Most men who suffer from impotence have a functional disorder of the "spongy" or erectile tissue in the penis. This erectile tissue is called the *corpus cavernosum*, and during a normal erection, it becomes congested with blood. If this congestion does not occur, the penis remains small and soft. New treatments available for this problem are vasoactive drugs such as alprostadil (also known as prostaglandin E_1 and sold under the name Prostin) that can be self-injected into the erectile tissue of the penis when required. These injections enable a man to regain control of his erections, although by artificial means. Most users of this method are very satisfied. If this fails, penile implants can be successful. For more detailed information about male impotence, I recommend the excellent and comprehensive book *It's Up to You* by Warwick Williams.[1]

ESTROGEN THERAPY FOR MEN

It used to be thought that the hormone estrogen exerted effects only on female sexual organs, such as the vagina, uterus, and breasts. We now know that estrogen exerts profound and widespread effects upon many other tissues, such as the brain, liver, bones, joints, skin, heart, and arteries. In particular, estrogen has a very favorable effect on blood cholesterol, as it helps the enzymes that break down cholesterol and thus reduces the chances of the blood vessels becoming blocked with plaque. In the long term, estrogen helps to reduce diseases of the heart and blood vessels.

This observation has led some of our modern-day scientists to come up with the hypothesis that if we give natural estrogen to males, we may be able to reduce their current high rate of cardiovascular disease. Indeed, there are now clinical trials underway to see if giving natural estrogen to men between the ages of thirty and sixty will reduce their cholesterol levels and incidence of heart attacks. Estrogen may also reduce the incidence of cancer of the prostate gland, so there may be several ways in which estrogen might give men an extra ten years or so of life.

All is not roses, however. Estrogen is a potent feminizing hormone, so it is likely to have some undesirable side effects for the male of the species. These could include breast tenderness, loss of sex drive, impotence, and reduced sperm production.

NUTRITIONAL STRATEGIES FOR "MALE MENOPAUSE"

Diet and lifestyle are supremely important for the man who finds himself with reduced mental and sexual performance during midlife.

Exercise is vitally important. However, given the current high rate of cardiovascular disease among men, I believe that all men should undergo a cardiac stress test (exercise EKG) before initiating an increase in their exercise program. A good age to have a cardiac stress test is forty to fifty—or even younger if there is a poor family history.

There are also some specific vitamins, minerals, herbs, and dietary supplements that can improve the functioning of the endocrine system, and in particular that of the testicles. Among the most important supplements for men in midlife are vitamin E, magnesium, zinc, ginseng, royal jelly, and the entire vitamin B complex. Table 9.1 provides an overview of these supplements, their functions, and recommended doses.

Vitamin E

I believe that all middle-aged men should take 500 international units of vitamin E (d-alpha-tocopherol) daily. Vitamin E is a superb antioxidant that is especially active in the *intima* (the inner layer of the arteries) and reduces atherosclerosis (hardening of the arteries) and heart disease. To remain sexually active and virile, you need healthy blood vessels to supply blood to the pelvic area.

Magnesium

Although sodium is the dominant mineral in today's oceans, the primordial oceans of the earth were rich in magnesium and potassium. The cytoplasm (intracellular fluid) in our bodies still resembles the "primordial soup" from which all forms of life arose. Our intracellular fluid is rich in the minerals magnesium and potassium, and our body works hard to maintain this state. Magnesium is found mainly in the bones, the muscles, and the fluid within our cells. It is vital for every important biological reaction, including the synthesis of protein and of genetic material, the metabolism of glucose, and the release of cellular energy.

Adequate magnesium is vital for a healthy cardiovascular system because it regulates nerve conduction, vascular tone, and the electrical stability of muscle cells, and it is essential for maintaining the integrity of cell membranes. Marginal magnesium deficiency is very common in many men, especially diabetics, regular drinkers, poor eaters, and those who exercise regularly and strenuously. Magnesium supplementation may reduce ischemic heart disease, cardiac arrhythmias, and cardiomyopathy. Good food sources of magnesium include seafoods, green vegetables, nuts, and low-fat dairy products. Recommended supplemental doses range from 250 to 800 milligrams of magnesium amino acid chelate daily.

Zinc

A daily 50-milligram zinc chelate supplement is most worthwhile for men. There is evidence that most of us become increasingly prone to zinc deficiency with age, and even in developed countries many men are at risk of marginal zinc deficiencies.

Zinc can increase male potency and libido, and may reduce prostate problems such as prostatitis (inflammation) and hypertrophy (enlargement). Also, gentlemen, it can reduce hair loss and aches and pains in the muscles and joints. However, you should be careful not to exceed the recommended dosage, as excessive amounts of zinc can cause stomach upset. Zinc is best taken intermittently—for example, three months on, three months off.

Ginseng

Ginseng is probably the most ancient and famous medicinal herb on earth. Its use in Chinese medicine dates back more than 4,000 years.

Soviet scientists began investigating ginseng in the mid-twentieth century, and found that it increased the body's resistance to a wide range of adverse factors.

There are two types of ginseng, Siberian (botanical name *Eleuthero-coccus senticosus*) and American (*Panax quinquefolius*). Better results seem to come from Siberian ginseng. Russian researchers claim that ginseng can boost immunity, inhibit cancer, and increase energy and stamina. Ginseng also enjoys a reputation as a "glandular tonic" for men, meaning that it improves testicular function.

Recommended doses range from 1,000 to 4,000 milligrams daily. However, ginseng should not be used by people with very high blood pressure (over 180/100).

Royal Jelly

This is the diet of the queen bee, and it is a potent mixture of pollen and special secretions from the glands of worker bees. It is a rich natural food containing vitamins, minerals, amino acids, and other nutrients. It is especially rich in choline, one of the precursors of acetylcholine, which is a neurotransmitter involved in sexual response and performance. Royal jelly has been used for centuries by the Chinese for its energy-boosting properties.

Vitamin B Complex

The B vitamins are essential for the normal functioning of the brain and peripheral nerves and thus for a healthy sex life. In particular, vitamin B_6 (pyridoxine), vitamin B_5 (pantothenic acid), and choline are needed for the manufacture of the neurotransmitters serotonin and acetylcholine. These neurotransmitters are vital for libido and for sexual performance and enjoyment. Acetylcholine is a memory-enhancing neurotransmitter and a balancer of the nervous system.

Many men and women, especially regular drinkers, are lacking some of the B vitamins, and would benefit by taking a vitamin B supplement. A good B complex tablet should contain vitamins B_1 (thiamine), B_2 (riboflavin), B_3 (nicain), B_5 (pantothenic acid), B_6 (pyridoxine), B_{12} (cyanocobalamin), and choline, and should be taken on a daily basis.

MALE MIDLIFE CRISIS

We know that, technically speaking, men cannot go through a literal

Table 9.1 Male Menopause Kit

There are a number of dietary supplements that can be extremely helpful for men in midlife. The following table outlines a suggested daily program of vitamins, minerals, and herbal supplements a man can use to improve his overall health and well-being.

Supplement	Daily Dose	Actions
Vitamin E	500 IU	As an antioxidant, vitamin E protects cell structures and reduces oxidative damage to the linings of blood vessels. Vitamin E also increases the efficiency of oxygen utilization by cardiac muscle and improves testicular function.
Minerals: • Magnesium • Zinc • Selenium • Manganese	500 mg 50 mg 50 mcg 5 mg	These minerals are antioxidants and work synergistically as catalysts for enzyme systems, increasing metabolic efficiency. Magnesium also improves cardiac function; zinc is helpful for symptoms of an enlarged prostate.
Ginseng and royal jelly	2,000–4,000 mg each	These are ancient "glandular tonics" used by Chinese and Russian civilizations. They boost energy and immunity.
Balanced vitamin B complex containing: • B$_1$ (thiamine) • B$_2$ (riboflavin) • B$_3$ (niacin) • B$_5$ (pantothenic acid) • B$_6$ (pyridoxine) • B$_{12}$ (cyano-cobalamin) • choline	1 tablet or capsule	The B vitamins are necessary for the efficient functioning of the central and peripheral nervous system. They are especially important for persons who are under stress or who consume excessive amounts of alcohol.
Evening primrose oil	3,000 mg	A good source of essential fatty acids, which improve the production and release of hormones (see page 136).

menopause. However, for many men midlife brings significant hormonal, physical, and psychological changes. Put these all together in a melting pot and you may very well have the ingredients for a male midlife crisis. This is undoubtedly one of the reasons why divorce rates soar at this time of life, and many women get the shock of their lives. Many women are left alone in their "empty nests" as their husbands flee the familiar domestic scene. Conversely, the male not infrequently gets the "nesting syndrome" and spreads his wings with a younger woman, finding that her youthfulness rekindles his feelings of manliness and passion, and feeling that life is beginning all over again. Of course, the women they leave behind can also get the "nesting syndrome" and run off with younger men. I see quite a few older women doing this and find it an interesting sociological phenomenon. And after all, women in general live longer than men do—six years longer overall, and nine to ten years longer for women who take natural estrogen at menopause—so to help a woman avoid loneliness in old age, a man ten years younger could probably fit the bill very nicely.

Usually, however, such situations are very emotional and can be extremely traumatic in the both the short and long term. Yet many of them could probably be averted if men received more information and supportive counseling, especially together with their wives, at this time in their lives. In some cases, the timely use of testosterone replacement therapy, even if only on a temporary basis, can put the sparkle back into a long-term sexual relationship.

A male who finds himself with symptoms of male menopause during midlife can be helped greatly either by hormone replacement therapy or by nutritional medicine and lifestyle changes. Yet many men feel ashamed to admit that they have lost their virility and prior energy and do not seek help. They either assume that no help is available, or they believe that it is unacceptable to complain of such symptoms lest they be seen as old or unmanly.

The female menopause is "out of the closet" today, and women feel comfortable talking about their experiences and expressing their needs. Men should follow suit, and not worry about fitting the old-fashioned stereotype of the macho male who never has (or at least never discusses) any problems or difficulties. Besides, it can be more character-building to "open up" and confront one's problems, and to acknowledge the need to change. Men needn't worry that this will make them less manly or attractive; indeed, many women tell me that they prefer the kind of men we call "snags"—"sensitive new-age guys."

Chapter 10

In Summary—
A Farewell Message
From the Author

When you arrive at menopause, there is no reason to fear a change of life for the worse. If you are well informed and aware of all your options, you have the tools to maintain, and even to improve, your quality and enjoyment of life. In fact, there is some evidence suggesting that the better informed you are, the less likely you are to suffer in the first place.[1]

Menopause is a time of learning and self-reappraisal. It is a time when you can take control of your life and shape its destiny. Above all, it is a time for taking pleasure in being a woman in your own unique style. And today, you have the opportunity to take advantage of the powerful benefits of preventative, nutritional, and herbal medicine; natural hormone replacement therapy; and an anti-aging plan, to help ease your transition. You can have confidence in yourself and your decisions, which should give you the persistence necessary to obtain the best care and treatment available. Whatever you choose, be it "designer HRT," orthodox medicine, nutritional or herbal medicine, Mother Nature, or a combination of any or all of these, you will be able to overcome any menopausal problems you may experience with accurate knowledge and a positive attitude.

You may go through occasional rough patches as you feel and see deep changes taking place in yourself. I hope that this handbook can serve you as a strong and meaningful lifeline at these times. Remember that I am feeling and understanding these changes with you, as are many of your sisters on this planet. If we can gain inspiration, hope, and love from each other, something very precious will have been achieved.

I have written this book because you and other women have

inspired and taught me so much, and I know that we can continue to inspire and teach each other for many years. I hope it helps you to enjoy your menopausal years and beyond. As far as I can see, this time of life can be the best ever!

Some Thoughts at Menopause

I have some lines in my face from fifty years of life.
They tell me of years in the sun, of sorrows and joys.
They tell me of time.
They tell me I have lived and that I am still alive.
They can't be erased. They can be softened. . . .
Do I long to be the smooth-skinned, freckle-faced kid I once was?
No. I long for the same thing today that I longed for then:
to be the best I am able to be.[2]

NOTES

Chapter 1
Menopause in a Nutshell

1. J.W. Studd et al., "Oestradiol and Testosterone Implants," *British Journal of Obstetrics and Gynaecology* 84 (1977): 314–315.

Chapter 2
The Long-Term Consequences of Estrogen Deficiency

1. M.J. Stampfer, G.A. Colditz, et al., "Postmenopausal Estrogen Therapy and Cardiovascular Disease," *The New England Journal of Medicine* 325 (11) (12 September 1991): 756–762.
2. Ibid.
3. R. Bergstrom, M. Falkeborn, I. Persson, et al., "Hormone Replacement Therapy and the Risk of Stroke: Follow-up of a Population-based Cohort in Sweden," *Archives of Internal Medicine* 153 (10) (24 May 1993): 1201–1209.

4. Brian Henderson, "An Epidemiological Evaluation of the Risks and Benefits of HRT," in *Proceedings of the Inaugural Scientific Meeting of the Australian Menopause Society* (Brisbane, Australia: Australian Menopause Society, September 1989).
5. Ibid.
6. Stampfer, Colditz, et al., "Postmenopausal Estrogen Therapy and Cardiovascular Disease."
7. F.S. Kaplan, "Osteoporosis: Pathophysiology and Prevention," in *Clinical Symposia*, Vol. 39 (1) (Ciba-Geigy Corporation, 1987), 1–32.
8. R.W. Smith, W.R. Eyler, and R.C. Mellingen, "On the Incidence of Senile Osteoporosis," *Annals of Internal Medicine* 52 (1960): 773–776.
9. N.S. Weiss et al., "Decreased Risk of Fractures of the Hip and Lower Forearm With Postmenopausal Use of Estrogen," *The New England Jour-*

nal of Medicine 303 (1980):
1195–1198.

10. Nelson B. Watts et al., "Intermittent Cyclical Etidronate Treatment of Postmenopausal Osteoporosis," *The New England Journal of Medicine* 323 (12 July 1990): 73–79.

11. M.W. Tilyard et al., "Treatment of Postmenopausal Osteoporosis With Calcitriol or Calcium," *The New England Journal of Medicine* 326 (1992): 357–362.

Chapter 4
Everything You Will Ever Need to Know About Hormone Replacement Therapy

1. J.W. Studd et al., "Oestradiol and Testosterone Implants," *British Journal of Obstetrics and Gynaecology* 84 (1977): 314–315.

2. J.C. Stevenson et al., "Effects of Transdermal Versus Oral Hormone Replacement Therapy on Bone Density in Spine and Proximal Femur in Postmenopausal Women," *Lancet* 336 No. II (1990): 265–269.

Chapter 5
The Most-Asked Questions About Menopause

1. Sandra Cabot, *The Body Shaping Diet Book* (New York: Warner Books, 1995).

2. R.D. Gambrell, Jr., "Oestro-

gen-Progestogen Replacement and Cancer Risk," *Hospital Practice* 15 (1990): 81–100.

3. B.K. Armstrong, "Oestrogen Therapy—Boon or Bane?" *Medical Journal of Australia* 148 (1988): 213–214.

4. K.K. Steinberg et al., "A Meta-analysis of the Effect of Estrogen Replacement Therapy on the Risk of Breast Cancer," *Journal of the American Medical Association* 265 (1991): 1985–1990.

5. Ibid.

6. A.H. MacLennan, for the Australian Menopause Society, "Consensus Statement. Hormone Replacement Therapy and the Menopause," *Medical Journal of Australia* 155 (1991): 43–44.

Chapter 6
Naturopathic Medicine for Menopause

1. K.D.R. Setchell et al., Nonsteroidal Estrogens of Dietary Origin: Possible Roles in Hormone-Dependent Disease," *American Journal of Clinical Nutrition* 40 (September 1984): 569–578.

   H. Adlercreutz, T. Fotsis, et al., "Determination of Urinary Lignans and Phytoestrogen Metabolites," *Journal of Steroid Biochemistry* 25 (5B) (November 1986): 791–797.

2. Barbara Evans, *Life Change* (London: Pan Books, 1979), 38.
3. R. Buist, "The Role of Nutrients in the Prevention of Heart Disease," report to the seminar "Nutrition in Disease Prevention," Sydney, Australia, Australian Council for Responsible Nutrition, 9 March 1992.
4. Ibid.

Chapter 7
Slowing Down the Aging Process

1. Ruth Cilento, *Heal Cancer* (Australia: Hill of Content, 1993).
   Lewis Harrison, *Making Fats and Oils Work for You* (Garden City Park, NY: Avery Publishing Group, 1990).
2. Daniel Rudman et al., "Effects of Human Growth Hormone in Men Over 60 Years Old," *The New England Journal of Medicine* 323 (1) (5 July 1990):1–6.
3. Ibid.

Chapter 9
Male Menopause— Fact or Fiction?

1. Warwick Williams, *It's Up to You* (Sydney, Australia: Williams & Wilkins, 1985).

Chapter 10
In Summary—A Farewell Message From the Author

1. Barbara Evans, *Life Change* (London: Pan Books, 1979), 38.
2. Kaylan Pickford, *Always a Woman* (New York: Bantam Books, 1982).

GLOSSARY

Adipose tissue. Fatty tissue.

Adrenal glands. Two small glands situated on top of the kidneys that secrete various hormones, including adrenaline, cortisone, and sex hormones.

Agoraphobia. Abnormal fear of open spaces. A person with severe agoraphobia will find it difficult or impossible to leave his or her home.

Anabolic steroids. Synthetic hormones that stimulate the growth of bone and muscle and have masculinizing effects on the body.

Androgen. Sex hormones that promote the development of masculine characteristics, such as facial and body hair.

Antioxidant. A substance that protects cellular structures against oxidative damage. Well-known antioxidants include vitamins A, C, and E; beta-carotene; the minerals zinc and selenium; and the enzyme superoxide dismutase (SOD).

Atrophy. Wasting or thinning of tissues or organs.

Autoimmune disease. Any of a group of diseases produced by an imbalance or malfunction of the immune system that causes the immune system to attack and inflame the body's own tissues and organs.

Cancer. A type of disease characterized by the rapid multiplication of abnormal cells, resulting in a malignant growth, or tumor, that may spread to and invade distant body parts.

Cancer chemotherapy. The administration of highly toxic chemical drugs into the body for the purpose of killing cancer cells.

Cardiovascular disease. Any disease of the circulatory system, which comprises the heart and blood vessels.

Cholesterol. A steroid classified as a lipid that is a constituent of all animal cells. High blood cholesterol levels increase the risk of cardiovascular disease. Dietary cholesterol is found in fats and oils of animal origin and in coconut oil.

Circulation. The recurrent movement of the blood through the various blood vessels of the body.

Collagen. A fibrous protein that gives elasticity and strength to the skin, bones, cartilage, and connective tissues.

Curettage. The procedure of surgically scraping a body cavity (such as the uterus) to remove tissue, blood, or abnormal growths.

Deficiency. Lack or insufficiency of an essential substance.

Dowager's hump. A forward-facing curve on the upper spine, below the neck, that forms as a result of compression of the spinal vertebrae.

Endocrine system. The network of ductless glands that manufacture and secrete hormones into the bloodstream, affecting the functioning of distant organs and tissues.

Endocrinology. The study and treatment of disorders of the glands and the hormones they secrete.

Endometrial ablation. A surgical procedure in which the inner lining of the uterus is destroyed by means of radio waves or a laser beam.

Endometriosis. A disorder in which endometrial cells, which are normally confined inside the uterine cavity, are scattered about outside the uterus, in the abdomen, and/or in the pelvic cavity. It usually results in pain, possibly severe pain, during menstruation.

Endometrium. The mucous membrane forming the inner layer or lining of the uterus.

Enzyme. Any of the many proteins that catalyze or facilitate chemical reactions in cells. They are necessary to break down, or metabolize, nutrients, drugs, and hormones.

Epidemiologist. A specialist who deals with the spread of diseases among populations.

Essential fatty acids. Fatty acids necessary for cellular metabolism that cannot be produced by the body but must be supplied in the diet.

Suitable sources are evening primrose oil, fish oil, and various seeds and nuts.

Estradiol. A natural estrogen found in the blood. It is the most potent of all the natural estrogens.

Estrogen. A sex hormone secreted primarily by the ovary that is responsible for female physical characteristics, such as the development of breasts and feminine curves, as well as for menstruation.

Estrogen receptors. Physical structures on the cell membranes that attract estrogen and responds to its effects.

Estrone. A natural estrogen found in the blood.

Fallopian tubes. The small tubes connected to the sides of the uterus, through which eggs pass from the ovaries to the uterus, and in which fertilization occurs.

Fibroids. Noncancerous growths in the uterus that consist of muscle and fibrous tissue.

Follicle-stimulating hormone (FSH). A hormone secreted by the pituitary gland that acts on the ovary, causing it to stimulate the development (ripening) of follicles (eggs). These follicles produce estrogen.

Frigidity. Sexual unresponsiveness in a woman.

Genetic engineering. Man-made alteration in the genetic structure of cells, usually done for breeding purposes, to eradicate diseases, or to enable cells to synthesize chemicals or hormones.

Gland. *See* Endocrine system.

Hereditary. The quality of being passed through the genes from parents to their offspring, as characteristics or diseases.

Hormone. Any of the many chemicals that are produced by various glands in the body and transported in the blood to affect distant cells and organs.

Hormone replacement therapy (HRT). The administration of hormonal preparations (natural or synthetic) to make up for the decline of natural hormone production by various glands.

Hypertension. High blood pressure.

Hypothalamus. A major control center of the brain that regulates temperature, appetite, thirst, and the function of hormonal glands. It is situated at the base of the brain and is directly connected to the pituitary gland.

Hysterectomy. Surgical removal of the uterus.

Implant. A chemical substance or object that is surgically implanted into a part of the body.

In vitro fertilization (IVF). Fertilization of the egg by the sperm outside of the body, in a laboratory environment.

Incontinence. The inability to restrain or control the discharge of urine or feces.

Inflammation. A condition characterized by swelling, redness, heat, and pain in any tissue. Inflammation may occur as a result of trauma, irritation, infection, or imbalances in immune function.

Insomnia. The inability to sleep.

Libido. Sexual desire.

Menopause. The final cessation of menstruation; the last menstrual period.

Menstruation. The cyclic (usually monthly) discharge of blood from the nonpregnant uterus; also called the menstrual period.

Metabolism. The complex of chemical processes utilizing the raw materials of nutrients, oxygen, and vitamins, along with enzymes, to produce energy for body functions.

Minerals. A group of inorganic substances that are essential for normal cellular metabolism and the maintenance of life.

Mucous membrane. A lubricating membrane lining an internal surface or an organ such as the intestines or genitourinary canal.

Naturopathic medicine. An approach to health care that emphasizes the prevention and treatment of illness with naturally occurring substances such as juices, vitamins, minerals, herbs, etc.

Osteoporosis. A disorder characterized by loss of bone mass due to loss of calcium and resulting in a porous condition of the bones; skeletal atrophy.

Ovaries. The female sex glands (gonads) located on each side of the uterus that produce eggs and sex hormones, including estrogen and progesterone as well as a smaller amount of androgens.

Palpitations. Irregular or rapid heartbeats.

Pap smear. A test in which cells are gently scraped from the cervix and smeared onto a glass slide for examination under a microscope. It is a screening test for cancer of the cervix.

Parathyroid hormone. A hormone secreted by the parathyroid glands that controls the body's calcium balance and metabolism.

Peak bone mass. The ultimate or maximum amount of bone in the skeleton, usually achieved around the age of thirty years.

Pelvic floor muscles. The muscles that form the anatomical "floor" of the pelvic cavity and give support to the pelvic organs, including the uterus, bladder, and rectum.

Perimenopausal. Referring to the years leading up to, during, and just after menopause (roughly ages forty-five to fifty-five).

Pharmacology. The science of drugs and their chemical structures, uses, and beneficial and adverse effects.

Pituitary gland. A mushroom-shaped gland that is connected by a stalk to the base of the brain. It manufactures many different hormones that in turn control other glands, such as the thyroid, the adrenal glands, and the ovaries.

Plethoric accumulations. Congestion with blood.

Postmenopause. The period of time after menopause.

Premenopause. The period leading up to menopause. Generally four to five years long, it usually starts in the late forties, but it can begin anytime after the age of thirty-five, and is characterized by hormonal imbalance.

Progesterone. A sex hormone secreted by the corpus luteum of the ovary that acts to prepare the uterus for the possibility of pregnancy.

Progestogen. A synthetic form of the hormone progesterone that is capable of producing menstrual bleeding.

Prolapse. The abnormal dropping or protrusion of a bodily organ or structure, most often the rectum (bowel), bladder, uterus, or vagina.

Recommended daily allowance (RDA). The daily intake of various nutrients recommended by government health authorities. Consumption of the RDA of vitamins and minerals should guarantee an adequate amount of nutrients to avoid deficiency under normal circumstances. However, for optimal health, many nutritionists recommend consuming more than the RDA of certain nutrients, especially vitamin E, vitamin C, and beta-carotene.

Sex hormone binding globulin (SHBG). A protein in the blood that binds with and transports the sex hormones estrogen, progesterone, and testosterone. When bound to SHBG, the sex hormones are inactive.

Stroke. A condition in which the blood supply to the brain is disturbed to the extent that normal brain function is interrupted. A stroke may be mild and transitory, with no lasting effects, or it may cause permanent brain damage resulting in any degree of disability or even death.

Testosterone. The primary sex hormone responsible for the development of masculine characteristics.

Thrombosis. The formation of a blood clot in a blood vessel.

Tubal ligation. A surgical sterilization procedure in which the fallopian tubes are cut and tied or pinched closed by the use of plastic rings or clips.

Uterus. The female reproductive organ in which the fertilized egg implants and develops into a baby; the womb.

Vagina. The genital cavity from the uterus to the vulva.

Vertebrae. The bone segments that form the spinal column.

Vitamins. A group of food factors essential for cellular metabolism and the maintenance of life.

Vulva. The external female genitalia.

BIBLIOGRAPHY

Adlercreutz, H., T. Fotsis, et al. "Determination of Urinary Lignans and Phytoestrogen Metabolites." *Journal of Steroid Biochemistry* 25 (5B) (November 1986): 791–797.

Armstrong, B.K. "Oestrogen Therapy—Boon or Bane?" *Medical Journal of Australia* 148 (1988): 213–214.

Asch, R.H., and R.B. Greenblatt. "Steroidogenesis in the Post-menopausal Ovary." *Clinics in Obstetrics and Gynaecology*, Vol. 4, No. 1 (April 1977): 85–106.

Australian Menopause Society. "Consensus Statement. Hormone Replacement Therapy and the Menopause." *Medical Journal of Australia* 155 (1991): 43–44.

Bergstrom, R., M. Falkeborn, I. Persson, et al. "Hormone Replacement Therapy and the Risk of Stroke: Follow-up of a Population-based Cohort in Sweden." *Archives of Internal Medicine* 153 (10) (24 May 1993): 1201–1209.

Buist, R. "The Role of Nutrients in the Prevention of Heart Disease." Report to the seminar "Nutrition in Disease Prevention." Sydney, Australia: Australian Council for Responsible Nutrition, 9 March 1992.

Cabot, Sandra. *The Body Shaping Diet Book.* New York: Warner Books, 1995.

Cordoza, Linda, et al. "The Effects of Subcutaneous Hormone Implants During the Climacteric." *Maturitas* 5 (1984): 177–184.

Evans, Barbara. *Life Change.* London: Pan Books, 1979.

Gambrell, R.D., Jr. "Oestrogen-Progestogen Replacement and Cancer Risk." *Hospital Practice* 15 (1990): 81–100.

Harrison, Lewis. *Making Fats and Oils Work for You.* Garden City Park, NY: Avery Publishing Group, 1990.

Henderson, Brian. "An Epidemiological Evaluation of the Risks and Benefits of HRT." *Proceedings of the Inaugural Scientific Meeting of the Australian Menopause Society.* Brisbane, Australia: Australian Menopause Society, September 1989.

Kaplan, F.S. "Osteoporosis: Pathophysiology and Prevention." *Clinical Symposia,* Vol. 39 (1). Ciba-Geigy Corporation, 1987.

MacLennan, A.H. "HRT Regimen for the Menopausal Woman." *Current Therapeutics,* March 1993: 43.

Rudman, Daniel, Axel Feller, et al. "Effects of Human Growth Hormone in Men Over 60 Years Old." *The New England Journal of Medicine,* 323 (1) (5 July 1990): 1–6.

Setchell, K.D.R., S.P. Borriello, P. Hulme, D.N. Kirk, and M. Axelson. "Nonsteroidal Estrogens of Dietary Origin: Possible Roles in Hormone-Dependent Disease." *American Journal of Clinical Nutrition* 40 (September 1984): 569–578.

Smith, R.W., W.R. Eyler, and R.C. Mellingen. "On the Incidence of Senile Osteoporosis." *Annals of Internal Medicine* 52 (1960): 773–776.

Stampfer, M.J., G.A. Colditz, W.C. Willett, et al. "Postmenopausal Estrogen Therapy and Cardiovascular Disease." *The New England Journal of Medicine* 325 (11) (12 September 1991): 756–762.

Steinberg, K.K., S.B. Thacker, et al. "A Meta-analysis of the Effect of Estrogen Replacement Therapy on the Risk of Breast Cancer." *Journal of the American Medical Association* 265 (1991): 1985–1990.

Stevenson, J.C., M.P. Cust, K.F. Gangar, T.C. Hillard, B. Lees, and M.I. Whitehead. "Effects of Transdermal Versus Oral Hormone Replacement Therapy on Bone Density in Spine and Proximal Femur in Postmenopausal Women." *Lancet* 336 No. II (1990): 265–269.

Studd, J.W., et al. "Oestradiol and Testosterone Implants." *British Journal of Obstetrics and Gynaecology* 84 (1977): 314–315.

Tilyard, M.W., et al. "Treatment of Postmenopausal Osteoporosis

With Calcitriol or Calcium." *The New England Journal of Medicine* 326 (1992) 357–362.

Watts, Nelson B., et al. "Intermittent Cyclical Etidronate Treatment of Postmenopausal Osteoporosis." *The New England Journal of Medicine* 323 (12 July 1990): 73–79.

Weiss, N.S., C.L. Ure, J.H. Ballard, A.R. Williams, and J.R. Daling. "Decreased Risk of Fractures of the Hip and Lower Forearm With Postmenopausal Use of Estrogen." *The New England Journal of Medicine* 303 (1980): 1195–1198.

RESOURCE ORGANIZATIONS

The following organizations offer a variety of services that may be of help to the menopausal woman. Be aware that addresses and telephone numbers are subject to change.

MENOPAUSE AND WOMEN'S HEALTH

A Friend Indeed
Box 1710
Champlain, NY 12919-1710
(514) 843–5730
Fax (514) 843–5681

Alliance for Aging Research
2021 K Street NW, Suite 305
Washington, DC 20006
(202) 293–2856

American College of Obstetrics
and Gynecology
409 Twelfth Street SW
Washington, DC 20024-2188
(202) 638–5577

Center for Climacteric Studies
University of Florida
901 NW Eighth Avenue, Suite B1
Gainesville, FL 32061

National Women's Health
Network
1325 G Street NW
Washington, DC 20005
(202) 347–1140

National Women's Health
Resource Center
2440 M Street NW, Suite 201
Washington, DC 20037
(202) 293–6045

North American Menopause
Society
University Hospitals
Department of Obstetrics/
Gynecology
2074 Abington Road
Cleveland, OH 44106
Fax (216) 844–3348
Written requests only.

Older Women's League (OWL)
666 Eleventh Street NW,
  Suite 700
Washington, DC 20001
(202) 783–6686

BREAST CANCER

National Alliance of Breast
  Cancer Organizations
1180 Avenue of the Americas,
  Second Floor
New York, NY 10036

National Cancer Institute
Cancer Information Service
9000 Rockville Pike
Bethesda, MD 20892
(800) 4–CANCER
(800) 422–6237

Y-ME
National Institute for Breast
  Cancer Information and
  Support
18220 Harwood Avenue
Homewood, IL 60430
(708) 799–8338

CARDIOVASCULAR DISEASE

American Heart Association
7320 Greenville Avenue
Dallas, TX 75321
(214) 373–6300

National Heart, Lung,
  and Blood Institute
9000 Rockville Pike
Bethesda, MD 20892
(301) 496–4236

OSTEOPOROSIS

National Osteoporosis Foundation
2100 M Street NW, Suite 602
Washington, DC 20037
(202) 223–2237

NUTRITION

American Dietetic Association
  (ADA)
216 West Jackson Boulevard,
  Suite 800
Chicago, IL 60606
(312) 899–0040

Center for Science in the
  Public Interest
1875 Connecticut Avenue NW,
  Suite 300
Washington, DC 20009-5728
(202) 332–9110

Index

Page numbers followed by (f) indicate figures; those followed by (t) indicate tables.

A MESSAGE FROM THE AUTHOR— DR. SANDRA CABOT, M.D.

I sincerely hope that you enjoyed this book and that you have found it useful in your own day-to-day life. There is so much to learn about our physical and mental well-being! Please feel free to write to me to give me feedback on this book or to make further inquiries.

From time to time I do seminars for women on menopause and other health-related topics. These give me an ideal opportunity to speak with individual women and to learn about their personal questions and concerns. If you feel you would be interested in attending one of my seminars, please write to me for information concerning my schedule. My address in the United States is:

Dr. Sandra Cabot
c/o Avery Publishing Group
120 Old Broadway
Garden City Park, NY 11040